Burns Trauma

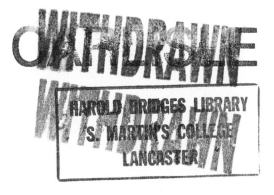
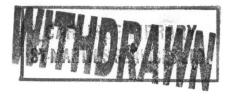
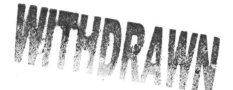
1873853327

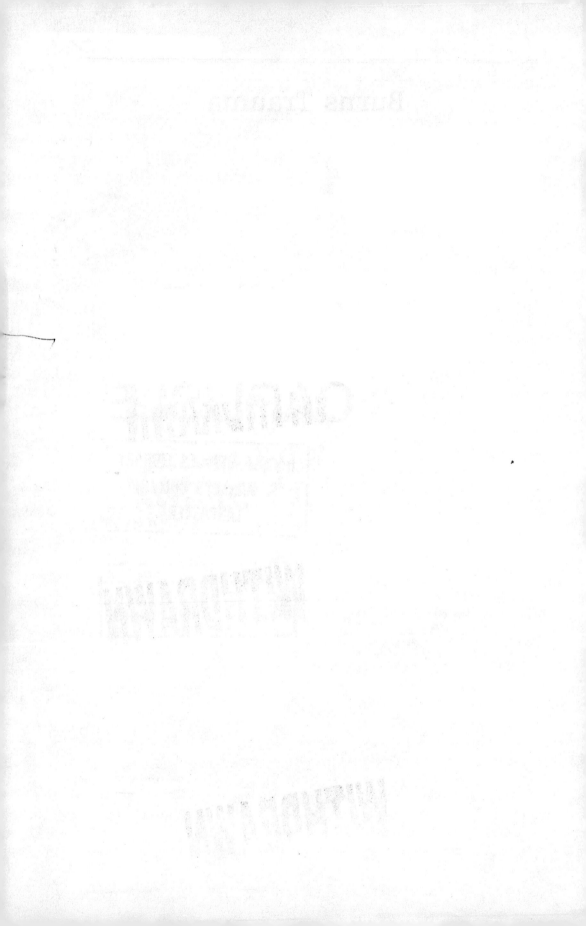

Burns Trauma
Management and Nursing Care

EDITED BY

Chrissie Bosworth
BSc (Hons) RGN
Clinical Nurse Specialist, Burns Unit
City Hospital NHS Trust, Nottingham

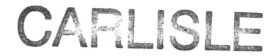
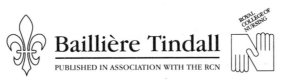

Baillière Tindall
PUBLISHED IN ASSOCIATION WITH THE RCN

London Philadelphia Toronto Sydney Tokyo

Baillière Tindall 24–28 Oval Road
London NW1 7DX

The Curtis Center
Independence Square West
Philadelphia, PA 19106-3399, USA

Harcourt Brace & Company
55 Horner Avenue
Toronto, Ontario, M8Z 4X6, Canada

Harcourt Brace & Company, Australia
30–52 Smidmore Street
Marrickville
NSW 2204, Australia

Harcourt Brace & Company, Japan
Ichibancho Central Building
Chiyoda-ku, Tokyo 102, Japan

A catalogue record for this book is available from the British Library

ISBN 1–873853–32–7

Typeset by Florencetype Ltd, Stoodleigh, Devon
Printed and bound in Great Britain by WBC, Bridgend, Mid Glamorgan

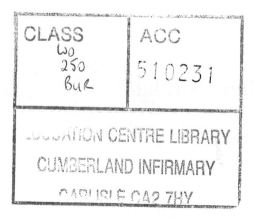

Contents

The colour plate section can be found between pages 116 and 117.

Contributors

Fiona Bailie, MB, BCh, BAO, FRCS, Ed, Consultant Plastic Surgeon, Burns and Plastic Surgery Unit, City Hospital NHS Trust, Nottingham

Deborah Beeby, RGN, RSCN, Dip. Health Studies, Senior Staff Nurse, Children's Unit, Peterborough District Hospital, Peterborough

Chrissie Bousfield (nee Bosworth), BSc (Hons), RGN, Nurse Teacher, School of Nursing and Midwifery, Faculty of Medicine and Health Science, University of Nottingham, Nottingham. Formerly Clinical Nurse Specialist, Burns Unit, City Hospital NHS Trust, Nottingham

Susan Boyle, RGN, Sister, Burns and Plastic Surgery Unit, Royal Preston Hospital, Preston

Deborah Cook, BSc(Hons), RGN, RNT, Nurse Practitioner, Northampton General Hospital NHS Trust, Northampton

Rosemary Gollup, Dip. Cot, SROT, Senior Occupational Therapist, Burns and Plastic Surgery Unit, Occupational Therapy Department, City Hospital NHS Trust, Nottingham

Gale A Harvey, RGN, Clinical Leader, Burns Unit, City Hospital NHS Trust, Nottingham

Owen C Jones, RNMH, RGN, Unit Manager, Burns Unit, City Hospital NHS Trust, Nottingham

Lisa Norman, BSc(Hons), SRD, Senior Paediatric Dietician, Nutrition and Dietetic Department, City Hospital NHS Trust, Nottingham

Sarah Pankhurst, RGN, Dip. Health Studies, Tissue Viability Nurse, Oak Tree Lane Health Centre, Nottingham

Stephen Regel, MA, RMN, Cert. Behav. Psycho, PGCe, Senior Lecturer in Health and Human Services, Department of Health and Human Services, Nottingham Trent University, Nottingham

Julie Spankie, MCSP, Senior Physiotherapist, Burns and Plastic Surgery, Physiotherapy Department, City Hospital NHS Trust, Nottingham

David Wilson, MB, BS, FRCS, Registrar, Burns and Plastic Surgery, Burns and Plastic Surgery Unit, City Hospital NHS Trust, Nottingham

Preface

Burn injuries, a unique form of trauma, are in many respects the worst injuries that an individual can experience (Wachtel et al, 1983). The management and nursing care of an individual following burn trauma is a specialised area that requires a wealth of knowledge and clinical skills from the members of a large multidisciplinary team.

The burn patient, during the course of the resulting injury, undergoes a variety of physical and psychological changes, and in order for members of the multidisciplinary team to effectively treat the patient and support the family, it is essential to have a clear understanding of the pathophysiological effects and the management required at each stage of recovery.

This book has been written as a resource for all grades of staff within the multidisciplinary team caring for patients of all ages with different types of burn injury, in a variety of clinical environments. Its aim is to increase the reader's understanding of the effects of burn trauma on the individual, and it outlines the management and care that will be required during the course of hospitalisation. It should also prove to be an additional resource for those nurses undertaking diploma- or degree-level nurse training and/or post-basic courses relating to the specialty of burn care.

Selected members of the multidisciplinary team with exceptional expertise in their clinical field have contributed chapters to provide a wide range of information, using a research-based approach and up-to-date references to ensure that our patients receive the high standards of care they deserve. I would like to acknowledge and thank all of the contributing authors who have shared their knowledge and clinical expertise. Without their contributions, this book would not exist.

Finally, I dedicate this book to all nurses who care for individuals who have sustained a burn injury, and especially to the burn patients themselves, facing the challenge of recovery from what must be a devastating experience in their lives.

Chrissie Bosworth

Reference

Wachtel TL, Kahn V and Frank HA (1983) Rehabilitation of the burn injured patient. *Current Topics in Burn Care*, pp 217–220: Rockville, MD: Aspen Systems Corporation.

Acknowledgements

Grateful thanks are extended to the Photographic Department and John Houghton, Staff Nurse on the Burns Unit at Nottingham City Hospital (NHS Trust) for their assistance in producing the illustrations in Chapters 6, 8, 10 and 12.

We are especially grateful for the generous financial assistance from the Nottingham City Hospital (NHS Trust), Burns and Plastic Surgery Charitable Funds, towards the publication of colour illustrations in the chapter on surgery.

We should also like to mention the helpful team at the Pressure Garment Manufacturing Unit of Camp Ltd, Long Eaton, and thank them for their kind contribution towards making the publication of this book possible.

Introduction

HISTORY OF BURN CARE

Ever since our ancestors discovered fire, man has knowingly risked his life to reap its benefits. This has inevitably led to accidental burn injuries, and many have paid the price of discovery with suffering, scarring and death (Kemble and Lamb, 1987).

In the writings of ancient Egypt and Greece (1600 BC), there are records of treating burns with oil-soaked cloths made from animal fat (Bryan, 1930). This may be considered as the ancient counterpart of the modern paraffin gauze dressing, which is still often used today. The Roman Empire (1st century AD) emphasised the use of herbs for wound therapy and even then practised surgical excision of contracted burn scars (Schumann, 1991).

There have been other major historical developments in the care of burns. In 1607, Hilanus described the three degrees of a burn, and in the 1800s Guillaume Dupuytren described six depths of burn injury. In 1897, the first saline solution infusions were given by Tommasoli in Sicily for fluid replacement in major burns, and in 1905, Wiedenfeld and Zumbush performed early wound excision within the first 3 days of a burn injury occurring (Haynes, 1987).

Underhill and associates in 1921 conducted a research study which demonstrated that burns shock was primarily a result of fluid loss during the initial burn period. Much of their research laid the foundation for modern fluid and electrolyte therapy, and served as a basis for further study into the pathophysiology of burns (Underhill et al, 1923).

The advent of skin grafting started with the techniques of the Swiss surgeon Reverdin, who performed the first epithelial graft in 1869 (Haynes, 1987), laying the foundation for modern split-thickness skin grafting (Schumann, 1991). However, the dermatome was not introduced until 1939 (Archambeault-Jones and Feller, 1981), and then prompted a move towards early wound closure and reduced mortality.

In 1954, Leidberg, Reiss and Artz discovered that septicaemia was a common cause of death in individuals following burn trauma (Leidberg et al, 1954) and this led to vigorous research on topical antimicrobial agents, which still continues today. Since then, advances in burn therapy have escalated dramatically. Half a century ago, an individual who had sustained burn trauma was one of the most neglected in surgery. Now, in specialised Burns Units, the patient is the object of keen competitive multidisciplinary care (Marvin, 1991).

The history of burn care would not be complete without mentioning Boston's Cocoanut Grove fire disaster of 1942, in which 492 lives were lost and hundreds of individuals were treated for burn injuries. This created a public movement for changes in building codes, building designs and standards of fire protection and prevention efforts, which are still prevalent today.

BURN PREVENTION/HEALTH PROMOTION

Burn prevention efforts have traditionally been directed at public education, and, despite numerous campaigns at international, national and local level, burn injuries continue to be a considerable health hazard for many people worldwide (Linares and Linares, 1990).

Many burn prevention campaigns are aimed at public education and increased awareness of burn safety, with behaviour modification as the ultimate goal. Some worldwide educational programmes undoubtedly have been successful in lowering burn injury rates and have been reported by Waller (1985), Herd et al (1986) and Keswani (1986).

However, these few successes notwithstanding, it is evident that after years of public education efforts, education alone has seldom resulted in a marked decrease in burn injuries. One important concept to consider is the attenuation effect that occurs normally from the implementation of an educational programme on prevention (McLoughlin et al, 1982).

Many research findings have documented the striking limitations of health education alone in motivating people to change their behaviour, and acknowledge that an increase in knowledge and awareness does not necessarily lead to a change in behaviour or lifestyle. Why then does health education have such little impact? The Health Belief Model formulated by Rosenstock (1974) and later modified by Becker et al (1974) helps to explain why some people follow recommended prevention measures while others do not. The Health Belief Model assumes that individuals are likely to take a health preventative action if, first, they believe they are susceptible to the injury, or that the injury could have serious effects on their life, second, they are aware of actions that can be taken and believe these actions may reduce the likelihood or severity of the injury, and, third, they believe that the threat to them of taking such action(s) is not as great as the injury itself.

An individual's subjective perception of contracting or encountering a specific health problem has been shown to be a strong indicator of taking preventative health actions (Janz and Becker, 1984). Thus, in the long term, increasing a person's perceived susceptibility to a burn injury may potentially lead to a change in behaviour, and when planning educational programmes directed at burn prevention, one may need to take motivational variables into account.

Motivation to change behaviour or to take a health action may be prompted by increasing an individual's perceived threat of a burn injury. For example, people may know it is dangerous to store flammable liquids in the garage, but if they do not perceive themselves or their family to be at risk or do not believe that a fire or explosion may result, they will, out of habit or a sense of 'it will not happen to me', continue with the practice. Therefore, it is important to modify an individual's perceived susceptibility to the injury (Linares and Linares, 1990).

We can no longer afford to implement educational programmes that have as their major goal an increase in knowledge and awareness. An approach that combines behaviour change, environmental control and product modification through education and legislation would be more likely to be successful in reducing the occurrence of burn injuries. Burn prevention campaigns involving education and legislation should be directed at changing behaviours through perceived susceptibility to burn injury and motivation to change behaviour, and environmental control and product modification, through public pressure and legislation (Linares and Linares, 1990).

The approach to burn prevention must be based on a solid knowledge of the aetiology of burn injuries, taking into account geographical variations and socio-economic backgrounds. Prevention methods must also be updated in response to current and changing causation factors.

Modification of products or environmental control can successfully reduce the incidence of certain burn injuries; for example, the Child and Young Persons Act (1914) makes it an offence if a child suffers a burn when there is no fireguard present. The Heating Appliances Act (1945/1971) and the Fireguards Act (1952) make it an offence to offer for sale new gas or electric fires not fitted with a fireguard to the safety standard of BSI specification BS 1945 (1971). The Nightdresses for Children Act (1962) makes it illegal to offer for sale children's nightdresses that are not flame resistant to BSI specifications BS 3121 (1967) and BS 5722 (1979) (Leveridge, 1991), However, there is still no legislation relating to children's pyjamas.

Product modification is also evident in the introduction of coiled kettle flexes designed to reduce the incidence of scald injuries caused by children pulling trailing electric flexes attached to kettles.

Modification of the environment, such as decreasing the hot water temperature to 130°F (54.4°C) or below, effectively lowers the risk of scald injuries, as it increases the exposure time for a full-thickness burn to occur (Feldman et al, 1978). Environmental control through the installation of smoke detectors should also effectively decrease house fire-related deaths.

Passive manoeuvres that protect the public through product modification, environmental redesign or control and legislation are generally more effective in preventing injuries than are active measures that depend on persistent long-term behavioural or lifestyle change. However, future efforts aimed at public education and promotion of legislation should continue, with the support of responsible authorities who understand the problems and authorise adequate funds to support them (Linares and Linares, 1990).

Health promotion appears to lend itself well to the domains of burn care, and in essence the burn is just the beginning. Health promotion is a positive team approach, and nurses and other members of the multidisciplinary team are in a unique position that allows them to assist individuals in promoting, protecting and maintaining their health care status during the course of recovery and rehabilitation.

THE BURN TEAM

The management and care of an individual following burn trauma has changed dramatically over the past 20 years, leading to decreased morbidity and improved survival, function and cosmetic results in the long term (Marvin, 1991). These changes have been accomplished by the dedication of a wide range of professionals working together as a multidisciplinary burn team.

Teamwork is an essential part of the management of the burn patient (Leveridge, 1991), and has proved to be effective in dealing with even the most complex patient senario. Although each member of the team – nurse, surgeon, anaesthetist, physiotherapist, occupational therapist, dietitian and psychologist – has a specific role, many of the roles overlap and require a co-ordination of activities to promote high-quality care and successful patient outcomes.

The nurse provides critical care, wound care and rehabilitation, promoting the return to activities of daily living. The role also involves giving emotional support to both the patient and the family, together with co-ordinating multidisciplinary team activities. The surgeon provides comprehensive medical/surgical care that promotes wound healing, while the anaesthetist directs anaesthesia for operative and major wound care procedures and co-ordinates the management of inhalation burn injuries. The roles of the physiotherapist and occupational therapist are to assist patients in regaining optimal physical function, and the dietitian is responsible for providing nutritional advice and support. The psychologist aims to improve patients' psychological and psychosocial well-being, as well as provide emotional support for the family and, additionally, members of the multidisciplinary team.

It is therefore evident that the management and care of the patient with a burn injury requires a unique body of knowledge and skills from a range of multidisciplinary team members, and encompasses a wide variety of roles and responsibilities.

To this end, the following chapters seek to provide a comprehensive text for a variety of professionals in different clinical settings, whether it is the Accident and Emergency Department, the Intensive Care Unit or the Burns Unit itself. The contents aim to outline burn trauma, methods of treatment and the overall management and care provided by members of the multidisciplinary team, while reflecting the philosophical foundation 'to provide and maintain high standards of care in an individual and family-centred environment'.

References

Archambeault-Jones CA and Feller I (1981) Burn care. Cited in: Kinney MR et al (1981) *ACCN's Clinical Reference for Critical Care Nursing*, pp 741–742. New York: McGraw-Hill.

Becker MH, Drachman RH and Kirscht JP (1974) A new approach to explaining sick role behaviour in low income populations. *American Journal of Public Health* **6:** 205.

Bryan CP (1930) *Ancient Egyptian Medicine. The Papyrus*. Ares, London: Ebers.

Feldman KW, Schaller TS, Feldman JA et al (1978) Tap water scald burns in children. *Paediatrics*, **62:** 1.

Haynes BW (1987) The history of burn care. Cited in: Beswick JA (1987) *The Art and Science of Burn Care*, pp 3–7. C. Rockville, Maryland: Aspen.

Herd AN, Widdowson P and Tanner NSB (1986) Scalds in the very young – prevention or cure? *Burns Journal* **12:** 246.

Janz NK and Becker MH (1984) The health belief model – a decade later. *Health Education* **11:** 1.

Kemble JVH and Lamb BE (1987) *Practical Burns Management*. London: Hodder & Stoughton.

Keswani MH (1986) The prevention of burning injury. *Burns Journal* **12:** 533.

Leidberg NC, Reiss E and Artz CP (1954) Infection in burns III. Septicaemia, a common cause of death. *Surgery, Gynecology and Obstetrics* **99:** 151.

Leveridge A (1991) *Therapy for the Burns Patient*. London: Chapman & Hall.

Linares AZ and Linares HA (1990) Burn prevention – the need for a comprehensive approach. *Burns Journal* **16:** 281–285.

McLoughlin E, Vince C, Lee AM et al (1982) Project burn prevention: outcome and implications. *American Journal of Public Health* **72:** 241.

Marvin J (1991) Cited in: Trofino RB (1991) *Care of the Burn Injured Patient*, pv. Philadelphia: FA Davis.

Rosenstock IM (1974). Historical origins of the health belief model. *Health Education Monograph* **2:** 328.

Schumann L (1991) History of burn care. Cited in: Trofino RB (1991) *Nursing Care of the Burn Injured Patient*, pp 3–7. Philadelphia: FA Davis.

Underhill EP et al (1923) Blood concentration changes in extensive superficial burns and their significance for systemic treatment. *Archives of International Medicine* **32:** 31.

Waller JA (1985) *Injury Control – a Guide to the Causes and Prevention of Burn Trauma*, pp 318–319. Lexington, Massachusetts: Lexington Books.

1

Pathophysiology of Burns

Burn trauma represents a major injury in terms of the physical and psychological damage to the individual. For the members of the multidisciplinary team to effectively treat the patient and support the family, an understanding of the pathophysiology of burn trauma is essential.

This chapter discusses the normal anatomy of the skin and the physiological responses that occur as a result of a burn injury.

NORMAL ANATOMY OF SKIN

Structurally, the skin consists of two principal parts: the outer, thinner epithelium called the **epidermis**, and the inner, thicker connective tissue part, the **dermis**. Beneath the dermis is a **subcutaneous** layer, which consists of areolar and adipose tissue (Figure 1.1).

The **epidermis** is organised into four or five cell layers, depending on its location in the body. Where exposure to friction is greatest, such as the palms and soles, the epidermis has five layers, whereas in all other areas it has four. The basement layer of cells divides and gradually sheds towards the surface. The cells lose their nuclei to become the dead horny keratin surface layer. A cell migrates from the basement membrane to the keratin layer in about 19 days. Passing through the epidermis are the hairs, secretion from the sebaceous glands and the ducts of the sweat glands.

The **dermis** is composed of connective tissue containing collagenous and elastic fibres. The dermis is very thick in the palms and soles and very thin in the eyelids, penis and scrotum. It also tends to be thicker on the dorsal aspects of the body than the ventral, and thicker on the lateral aspects of extremities than the medial. Numerous blood vessels, lymphatics, nerves, glands and hair follicles are embedded in the dermis. The sweat glands, sebaceous glands and hair follicles are derived from the epidermis, growing down into it during embryonic development. The combination of collagenous and elastic fibres in the dermis provides the skin with strength, extendibility and elasticity. The ability of the skin to stretch can readily be seen in pregnancy, obesity and oedema.

The dermis is attached to underlying organs, such as bone and muscles, by the subcutaneous layer. Beneath the dermis is a plexus of capillaries and the subdermal layer of fat.

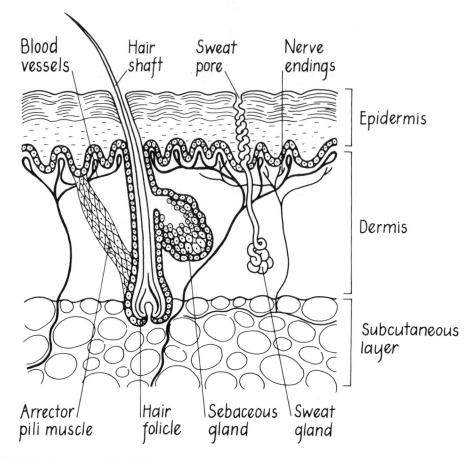

Fig 1.1 Anatomy of the skin

FUNCTIONS OF SKIN

For the average adult, the skin occupies a surface area of approximately 1.8 m². The skin is quite complex in structure and serves several functions essential for survival.

Maintenance of Body Temperature

The body temperature is normally maintained at an average of 36.8°C. If the temperature is raised, metabolism increases, and if it is lowered, metabolism decreases. The skin helps to ensure that a fine balance is maintained between heat produced by the body and heat lost to the environment, 97% of heat loss from the body being via the skin.

The amount of heat lost from the skin depends to a great extent on the amount of blood in the vessels in the dermis. As the amount of heat produced by the body increases, the arterioles become dilated, and more blood pours into the capillary network in the skin. In addition to increasing the amount of sweat produced, the temperature of the skin rises. When this happens heat is lost by:

- *Radiation* – exposed parts of the body allow heat to radiate away into the environment (providing the air temperature is below surface body temperature)
- *Conduction* – the clothes in contact with the body carry heat away
- *Convection* – the air passing over the exposed parts of the body and clothing carries heat away with the rising current
- *Evaporation* – sweat is discharged onto the skin surface and evaporates

Protection

The skin protects the deeper and more delicate organs and acts as the main barrier against the invasion of micro-organisms and other harmful agents.

The sebaceous glands pour their secretion, **sebum**, into the hair follicles and onto the skin. Sebum provides some waterproofing, keeps the skin soft and pliable, acts as a bactericidal agent to prevent the successive invasion of micro-organisms, and prevents drying, especially on exposure to heat and sunshine.

Melanocytes in the basement layer of skin react to ultraviolet radiation by the production of the pigment **melanin**, which absorbs ultraviolet rays.

Perception of Stimuli

The skin contains numerous nerve endings and receptors that detect stimuli related to temperature, touch, pressure and pain. Owing to the presence of the sensory nerve endings, the body reacts by reflex action to unpleasant or painful stimuli, and thus protects itself from further injury.

Fluid and Electrolyte Balance

Intact keratin is nearly waterproof, whereas dermis denuded of epidermis is permeable. Except via glandular secretion, little or no fluid, protein or electrolytes pass through intact skin. However, copious sweating will cause loss of sodium and chloride ions, as well as water.

Synthesis of Vitamin D

Ultraviolet light from sunlight converts 7-dehydrocholesterol in the skin into vitamin D. It is used with calcium and phosphorus in the formation and maintenance of bone. Excess of requirements is stored in the liver.

LOCAL PATHOLOGY

Burn injury to the skin deranges its functions and causes the following patho-physiological changes:

1. When damage is small, such as light sunburn, capillaries in the dermis become widely dilated, resulting in redness. Some fluid loss from the capillaries into the tissues may cause a rise in interstitial tissue pressure, stimulation of nerve endings and pain.

2. In a more severe burn, the fluid loss from the capillaries accumulates as blisters, either within the dermis or at the junction of the dermis and epidermis. The overlying epidermal cells die and must be regenerated from adjacent epithelium.

3. When a burn destroys the upper part of the dermis in addition to the epidermis, regeneration has to take place from epithelial elements in the glands and hair follicles. This can take 10–14 days.

4. A more severe injury will destroy the dermis, leaving a few epithelial remnants in glands and hair follicles only in the subdermal fat layer. Deep dermal burns will only re-epithelialise slowly, resulting in poor, thin skin.

5. Destruction of all skin elements may also burn underlying muscle, bone or tendon. This type of burn injury will not heal without surgical intervention.

Circumferential burns may compromise blood supply to the limbs or breathing if the neck/chest are involved.

SYSTEMIC PATHOPHYSIOLOGY

Burn injury can destroy the proteins in the exposed cells and cause cell injury or death. The injury to tissues directly or indirectly in contact with the damaging agent, such as the skin or the linings of the respiratory and digestive tracts, is the local effect of the burn. Generally, however, the systemic effects of a burn are a greater threat to life than are the local effects. The systemic effects of a burn may include the following:

Cardiovascular Effects

Reduction in the volume of blood in active circulation is a common denominator in shock, and the central role of hypovolaemia in burns shock was emphasised by Blacock in 1931. However, it was not until the 1940s that the magnitude of the fluid shift in burns began to be elucidated (Cope and Moore, 1947). Prior to that, it was thought that the only loss of plasma from the circulation was that which could be seen leaving the surface of the burn wound.

Within minutes of a burn being sustained, oedema begins to gather beneath the damaged areas, a result of changes in capillary permeability in tissues affected, but not devitalised, by heat. The development of this oedema appears to be obligatory; as yet no treatment has been found that will stop the plasma leak from the affected vessels. The amount of oedema that occurs depends partly upon the circumstances of the burn, i.e. the temperature and the time of exposure, and partly upon the elasticity and tissue tension of the area affected. Thus, in the face, where the tissues are relatively lax and easily distensible, the swelling will be great and obvious, while in places with a high tissue elasticity, such as the limbs, much less swelling will occur (Muir et al, 1987).

The composition of the burn oedema is essentially that of plasma but with rather less protein. This is due to the dilutional effect of fluid drawn from the uninvolved interstitial compartment. The oedema continues to accumulate until a new balance is struck between the intravascular and extravascular compartments (Arturson, 1979).

This leakage is maximal in the first 8 hours after the burn, and then gradually decreases until, after 48 or 72 hours, the patient creates more fluid in their circulatory system, has a diuresis and becomes more physiologically stable (Pruitt and Mason, 1971; Pitt et al, 1987). This timing varies at either end of the age scale, being quicker to settle in younger patients, and the process is slower in deeper, larger burns.

In a burn of up to 30% body surface area, the leakage is around the injured area, but when it is over 30%, the leakage becomes generalised. The loss of plasma from the capillaries leads to haemoconcentration, i.e. an increase in the ratio of red cells to plasma in the blood. The blood becomes more viscous, and circulation in the capillaries may be slowed or stopped. Because of poor tissue perfusion, the depth of the burn will be increased as a result of lack of oxygen supply to the tissues.

Without treatment, the haematocrit will progressively rise; by the time one half of the plasma volume has been lost into the burn, the haematocrit will be between 60 and 70%. One-third of the total blood volume will then have been lost, the signs and symptoms of severe shock will be present, and the patient's life will be in danger. Without treatment, an individual with an extensive burn (over 50% body surface area) reaches this stage within 3–4 hours of the accident.

The loss of this protein-rich fluid from the plasma at the site of the burn is the factor of overriding importance in the causation of the clinical condition of shock in burned patients.

Signs and Symptoms of Shock

The signs and symptoms of shock vary with the severity of the condition, but the following signs are characteristic:

1. Hypotension, in which the systolic blood pressure is lower than 90 mmHg, owing to generalised vasodilatation and decreased cardiac output.

2. Cool, clammy, pale skin, owing to vasoconstriction of the peripheral circulation, and sweating as a result of sympathetic stimulation and increased adrenaline levels.

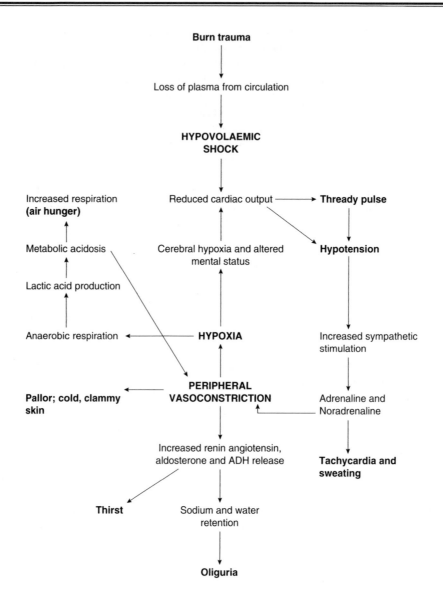

Fig 1.2 Pathophysiology of shock

3. Reduced urine output, inadequate for effective clearance of waste products normally dealt with by the kidney, because of hypotension and increased levels of aldosterone and ADH.

4. Altered mental status, owing to cerebral ischaemia. The patient may initially be alert and apprehensive, but as shock progresses, becomes disturbed, disorientated and restless to an extreme degree. Consciousness may only be lost as a pre-terminal event.

5. Weak, thready pulse as a result of generalised vasodilatation and reduced cardiac output, with little evidence of capillary filling. There is also tachycardia, owing to sympathetic stimulation and increased levels of adrenaline.

6. Thirst, owing to loss of extracellular fluid. Administration of fluids by mouth usually produces vomiting.

7. Breathing is at first rapid and shallow, but later becomes gasping and is described as air hunger. Acidosis results from the build-up of lactic acid.

It is essential to realise that all of these features are the result of inadequate perfusion of the body tissues. They are evidence of compensatory mechanisms, both reflex and hormonal, that serve to maintain blood flow to the cerebral and coronary vessels until the last possible moment. There is no treatment for them other than restoration of the circulation (Figure 1.2).

Following a major burn injury, cardiac output falls within half an hour or so to one-third of normal. This initial fall is obligatory and is unaffected by rapid transfusion (Horton et al, 1989). However, transfusion to replace circulating fluid volume can prevent or reduce a later fall in cardiac output from 6–8 hours post-injury. The initial fall is thought to be due to factors released into the plasma (Raffa and Trunkey, 1978). As fluid therapy is administered, cardiac output progressively returns to normal or above by 24–36 hours.

Red blood cells undergo changes after a burn injury. There is an immediate haemolysis in the region of the burn, and, if the quantity destroyed is sufficient, this will manifest as obvious haemoglobinaemia and haemoglobinuria. However, red cells additionally have a reduced life span, becoming abnormally fragile and being removed by the reticuloendothelial system, so that the haemoglobin level may fall markedly within a few days of injury (Muir et al, 1987).

Transfused blood will undergo the same haemolysis as the patient's own cells, and may increase the already elevated blood viscosity, leading to further impairment of the microvascular flow. The white cell count is usually raised following a burn injury, but function is poor, reducing resistance to infection.

Kidney, Fluids and Electrolytes

After a severe burn, under the action of angiotensin, catecholamines and the anti-diuretic hormones of the posterior pituitary, renal blood flow and urine output diminish (Le Quesne, 1957), and acute tubular necrosis may follow inadequate fluid replacement. In deep burns affecting muscle or bone – typically high-voltage electrical burns – myoglobinuria or haemoglobinuria may be present owing to the destruction of erythrocytes or muscle blocking tubules giving a pigmented urine. Unless treated, this can lead to rapid renal failure.

Glycosuria occurs in individuals with large burns as part of the stress response owing to depletion of pancreatic insulin. This pseudo-diabetes usually lasts for up to 48 hours, is unaccompanied by symptoms and is differentiated from true diabetes by the absence of ketones in the urine and by a glucose tolerance test (Bailey, 1966).

The large volumes of fluid that move from one compartment to another in burns shock are associated with corresponding shifts of electrolytes. Damaged collagen in the burned area selectively absorbs sodium, and the membranes of damaged cells allow sodium to leak into the cells and potassium to leak out. Hypokalaemia may be severe enough to warrant replacement therapy.

Pulmonary Changes

The incidence of pulmonary complications associated with a burn injury is approximately 22%, but the mortality of this group is of the order of 80% (Achauer et al, 1973). Initial lung damage may occur from the inhalation of hot gases, from irritants such as smoke or from anoxia.

The upper airway, nasal passages, mouth, pharynx and trachea respond by the formation of oedema, which may continue for up to 48 hours, leading to obstruction of the airway. The bronchioles and alveoli also become oedematous, and perfusion becomes inadequate. Acidosis may ensue as carbon dioxide is not cleared.

As airway oedema subsides, over 3–4 days after the injury, increased mucus production and a reduction in cilial activity combine to increase the risk of infection. Debris becomes detached from the small airways, which then become obstructed, adding to the increased shunt fraction seen following major burns.

Adult respiratory distress syndrome (ARDS) is well described in association with major burn injury, possibly due to mediators released from the burn or resulting from an inhalation injury damaging the pulmonary capillary endothelial membrane.

Ventilation may also be hampered by encircling eschar around the chest or neck, by the outpouring of transudate into the alveolar spaces and by elevation of the diaphragm by an intestinal ileus.

Metabolic Effects

Large quantities of heat may be lost from the burned patient as a result of:

● Loss of the thermoregulatory function of damaged skin
● Increased evaporation of fluid from the weeping burn

Under the abnormal conditions of additional water loss in a burned patient, heat loss may exceed body heat production, unless additional energy is supplied in the form of a high ambient room temperature (up to 28°C or more) and additional calories from nutrition.

In the healthy body, protein synthesis and breakdown are in equilibrium. In the burned patient, synthesis is usually normal but breakdown is greatly accelerated. This is shown by an increase in urinary urea and creatinine.

Gastrointestinal Tract Effects

The early vomiting often experienced when giving oral fluids to the recently burned patient is the result of gastric dilatation and intestinal ileus owing to splanchnic vasoconstriction, and may occur several days after the burn injury. It may be associated with electrolyte imbalance and is also a sign of sepsis.

Unexplained hypotension, haematemesis or melaena may result from ulceration of the gastrointestinal tract, usually from multiple points. Gastric perforation is more likely with larger burns and can occur some 10–14 days after injury. This is the ulcer that was described by Curling in 1842 and is usually known by his name.

Endocrine Sequelae

Burn injury is associated with a marked endocrine response (Dolecek, 1989). Catecholamines and cortisol are raised, and impaired glucose tolerance is a common feature.

Immune function is suppressed more in burned than other trauma patients, rendering them highly susceptible to infection. Various immunosuppressive factors have been isolated from burn serum; they may originate from burn tissue or be released by an intense local inflammatory response following severe burn injury (Hansborough et al, 1990).

Endotoxin, released from macrophages, elicits the production of tumour necrosis factor (TNF), which causes coagulopathy, shock, fluid and electrolyte sequestration and widespread organ damage, and is in itself a pyrogen. The resetting of the hypothalamic thermostat will make the patient pyrexial, usually at 38–39°C (Marano et al, 1990).

PATHOPHYSIOLOGY OF ELECTRICAL BURNS

The pathophysiology of electrical injury may appear mild when viewed as only local pathology, but the severity of the damage may be much worse systemically. Electrical current enters the body at the point of contact, travels along planes and structures of low resistance, and exits through the earth contact.

Only the contact points initially produce visible skin injury. Factors that influence the amount of tissue damage include:

1. *Voltage* High-tension voltages ionise the air particles and may arc across several metres (making physical contact with the electrified victim unnecessary for the sustaining of injury). Voltages as small as 45 volts have been fatal.

2. *Amperage*   Current determines the heat generated. Ventricular fibrillation has been induced by 100 amps on the heart, and the effect of amperage is related to the length of time it is applied.

3. *Resistance*   In ascending order of resistance, blood vessels, nerves, muscles, skin, tendon, fat and bone provide a pathway for passage of the current. Thrombosis of blood vessels may result in ischaemic or venous gangrene of tissue supplied by those vessels, at some distance from the burn injury. Skin immersed in water has a reduced resistance, compared with dry skin.

Damage is produced by:

● Heat from the passage of the current through tissue
● Damage to vessels, producing ischaemic necrosis
● Interference with electrical conductivity of organs, such as the heart and nerves
● Tetanic contraction of muscle
● Thermal injury from ignition of clothing
● Forceful propulsion of the body, producing spinal or limb fractures and intraperitoneal and intrathoracic injury

Unexplained hypokalaemia may occur within a few hours of injury and persist for several weeks. This may be explained by alteration of the cell membrane potential caused by the electrical injury, affecting electrolyte exchange across the cell wall.

Burning by contact with electrical current that passes through the body has effects upon the heart, brain, abdominal cavity, muscles, blood vessels and nerves. In addition, it destroys the skin that comes into contact with the electrical source. For this reason, the estimation of the extent of the burn by measuring the percentage body surface area of the burn is valueless. Considerably greater quantities of tissue may be destroyed beneath intact skin than is superficially apparent.

References

Achauer BM, Allyn PA, Furnas DW et al (1973) Pulmonary complications of burns; the major threat to the burn patient. *Annals of Surgery* **177:** 311–319.

Arturson G (1979) Microvascular permeability to macromolecules in thermal injury. *Acta Physiologica Scandinavica* **463** (suppl.): 111.

Bailey BN (1966) Hyperglycaemia in burns. *British Medical Journal* **2:** 1783.

Blacock A (1931) Experimental shock. VIII. The importance of the local loss of fluid in the production of the low blood pressure after burn. *Archives of Surgery* **22:** 610.

Cope O and Moore FD (1947) The redistribution of body water and the fluid therapy of the burned patient. *Annals of Surgery* **126:** 1010.

Dolecek R (1989) Endocrine changes after burn trauma – a review. *Keio Journal of Medicine* **38:** 262–276.

Hansborough JF, Zapata-Sirvent R and Hoyt D (1990) Postburn immunosuppression: an inflammatory response to the burn wound? *Journal of Trauma* **30:** 671–675.

Horton JW, Baxter CR and White DJ (1989) Differences in cardiac responses to resuscitation from burn shock. *Surgery, Gynecology and Obstetrics* **168:** 201.

Le Quesne LP (1957) *Fluid Balance in Surgical Practice*, 2nd edn. London: Lloyd-Luke.

Marano MA, Fong Y, Moldawer LL et al (1990) Serum cachectin/tumour necrosis factor in critically ill patients with burns correlates with infection and mortality. *Surgery, Gynecology and Obstetrics* **170:** 32–38.

Muir IFK, Barclay TL and Settle JAD (1987) *Burns and their Treatment*, 3rd edn. London: Butterworth.

Pitt RM, Parker JC, Jurkovich GJ et al (1987) Analysis of altered capillary pressure and permeability after thermal injury. *Journal of Surgical Research* **42:** 693.

Pruitt BA and Mason AD (1971) Haemodynamic studies of burned patients during resuscitation. In: *Research in Burns: Transactions of the Third International Congress on Research in Burns*, pp. 42–48. Bern, Switzerland: Hans Huber.

Raffa J and Trunkey DD (1978) Myocardial depression in acute thermal injury. *Journal of Trauma* **18:** 90–93.

2
Classification of Burns

Rarely does a week go by without reports of the death of one or more people involved in a house fire. Although serious burns are less common than minor ones, they are an important cause of mortality and morbidity. In England and Wales during 1988, 900 people died from the effects of fire, and 15 000 required admission to hospital (Wardrope and Smith, 1992). A much larger number of patients are managed in Accident and Emergency Departments: approximately 150 000 new patients will attend these departments each year with a burn injury, many of whom represent smaller, usually superficial, burns (Westaby, 1989). This chapter looks at the causes of burn trauma and the methods of classifying injuries according to their depth and percentage body surface area. Severity of injury and related mortality are also discussed.

Although burns injuries are often unpredictable, particular patterns to burn accidents can be identified in specific age groups. Under the age of 3, scalds predominate, most happening in or near the kitchen or bathroom. Some 70% of superficial burns occur in children under 5 years, with a peak incidence at 1–2 years, when children have attained both mobility and curiosity without having achieved caution. From age 3 to age 14, most injuries are due to clothes catching fire, or are the result of conflagration. From 15 to 60 years old, industrial accidents predominate, while after the age of 60, the general effects of ageing result in an increased risk of thermal injury (Dyer and Roberts, 1990). Abuse of cigarettes, drugs and alcohol is frequently responsible for the more serious complications of burns in the adult population. In almost all age groups, there are proportionally more burn injuries to males than females. Boys are frequently burned while experimenting with chemicals and fireworks, or by grabbing onto high-tension cables when climbing. Young girls are often burned while helping in the kitchen.

The type of injury varies according to factors such as the rural or industrial nature of the environment and the predominant type of heating in the homes. The majority of fire casualties occur in houses, as do scald injuries to children, which occur almost exclusively in homes. Only 18% of non-fatal and 10% of fatal fire injuries occur in buildings such as factories, hotels, schools and restaurants. Cooking appliances left on or unattended are responsible for starting 35% of all home fires and account for 27% of non-fatal and 6% of fatal casualties. More devastating still are cigarettes, cigars, pipe ash and matches, which are responsible for 28% of non-fatal and 39% of fatal casualties. Heating appliances, such as electric and gas fires and heaters, lead to 13% of non-fatal and 19% of fatal casualties (Harvey Kemble and Lamb, 1987).

TYPES OF BURN

There are several types of burn injury:

1. *Scalds* – injury from hot fluids such as tea, coffee, bathwater and saucepan contents. Although most scalds result in superficial skin loss, boiling water from a domestic kettle will cause full-thickness skin loss in a few seconds. Steam will cause greater damage, owing to the release of the latent heat of vaporisation. Boiling fat is at a higher temperature, and deeper damage results.

2. *Flame* – ignition of clothing from unguarded gas and electric fires, matches, open coal fires and explosion of paraffin and petrol-ignited bonfires or barbecues. In the elderly, a cigarette dropped into the armchair or bedclothes is all too often fatal. Burns from clothing that has caught fire are almost always serious. *Flash* burns occur when skin is momentarily exposed to high temperatures, for example lightning.

3. *Chemical* – from napalm and phosphorus used in military combat, bleaches, domestic cleaners, industrial acids and alkalis, agricultural lime and cement. Cytotoxic drugs injected extravenously by accident can produce extensive tissue necrosis. The severity of the burn will depend on the type of chemical, its concentration and the contact time.

4. *Electrical* – high-tension overhead or underground power cables carry 32 000 or more volts. Contact with the cable may be accompanied by violent propulsion of the patient in the explosion, causing fractures or intraperitoneal bleeding. High-voltage supply will cause severe and extensive burns with massive tissue destruction. Domestic burns (240 volts a.c.) occur when a live terminal or wire is touched while the patient is earthed.

5. *Radiation* – the most common burns of this nature are those caused by exposure to sunlight or sunbeds; they are usually superficial. They may also result from inadvertent escape of nuclear fuels, accidents during radiotherapy or the deliberate use of destructive weapons. These wounds are slow to heal because of the induced thromboangitis, and the resulting scar tissue is prone to further ulceration.

6. *Contact* – with hot metals, domestic appliances, such as irons or ovens, and bitumen. Contact with extreme cold temperatures, as in frost bite, is another cause. *Friction* burns may result from road traffic or other accidents resulting in shearing of the skin against another surface.

7. *Inhalation* – of hot gases or smoke, usually when the incident occurs within a confined space. Inhalation injury greatly increases the risk of mortality.

ABUSE

Abuse is the cause of many thermal burns in children (Purdue et al, 1988). A careful social history may reveal abuse in other family members or previously unexplained injuries to the victim. Risk is increased for male children, less than 3 years of age, who are left alone with a babysitter or boyfriend, although women also may abuse children. A delay in seeking medical attention for the child of more than 30 minutes after the injury should raise the question of abuse (Hobbs, 1986). Specific patterns of injury have also been identified. Circular burns from cigarettes and scald injuries with sharply defined margins, especially in a stocking or glove distribution, must be suspect. Perineal burns in children who are not yet toilet trained should always be reported as possible abuse (Purdue et al, 1988).

DEGREE OF INJURY

The depth of burn will depend on (Dyer, 1988):

- The *intensity/concentration* of the burning agent
- The *time* the agent is in contact with the skin

When patients are first seen, an attempt should be made to assess the depth of the burn injury. Describing the injury as a first-, second- or third-degree burn can be misleading, as these terms do not have a uniform meaning. It is less liable to cause misunderstanding if descriptive terms are used.

The most important aspect of the depth of the burn is whether or not the skin has been destroyed in its entire thickness, and it is this distinction that should be attempted during early assessment (Table 2.1). When the burned areas are mapped out on a body outline chart, some simple form of shading should indicate which parts are thought to be full thickness skin destruction and which parts only partial thickness skin damage.

Unfortunately, there is no simple test that will enable this distinction to be made with certainty on all occasions. However, it is usually well worth while testing the burned areas for sensation to pinprick. If the patient feels pain when the skin is pricked firmly with a sterile needle, viable cells must be present, and the burn is of partial thickness (Jackson, 1953). The majority of flash burns and scalds are of this type. Burns from blazing clothing – particularly when saturated with paraffin or petrol – which are dark brown, leathery hard and show evidence of thrombosed veins, are obviously full thickness skin destruction and are analgesic to needles and scalpels.

Some burns and scalds have a mottled red and white appearance, with a moist surface from which the most superficial layers of the skin have been lost or removed. These burns are quite often analgesic to pinprick, yet are capable of re-epithelialisation from epithelial elements surviving in the deepest parts of the

Table 2.1 Characteristics of burns
(Reproduced from Kemble and Lamb, 1987, with permission)

	Partial thickness	**Full thickness**
Length of contact with burning agent	Momentary	More than a few seconds
Temperature of burning agent	40–55°C	Boiling water, hot metal
Electrical injury	Unlikely	Probable
'Flash' burn without contact	Probable	Possible
Soles of feet and back of trunk	Probable	Possible
Amount of pain in burn	Painful	Painless
Appreciation of sharpness to pinprick test	'Sharp'	Appreciates touch or anaesthesia
Pressure on burn with forceps	Blanches	No change
Removal of forceps	Circulation returns	No change
Circulation in subcutaneous veins	Present	Absent, thrombosed
Appearance	Pink, blistering	White or charred

Table 2.2 Clinical depth of burn
(Reproduced from Kemble and Lamb, 1987, with permission)

	History	**Appearance**	**Blisters**	**Sensation**	**Result**
Superficial	Momentary exposure or sunburn	Red, bloated	Absent	Painful	Heals in approximately 7 days
Partial Thickness	Scalds of limited duration	Red or pink, with capillary return	Present, or surface wet or waxy	Painful	Heals in approximately 14 days
Full Thickness	Contact with high temperature or chemicals, or electrical injury	Charred, brown or white, dry thrombosed vessels	Absent	Painless	Granulates

sweat glands and hair follicles. It can be seen then that sensation to pinprick is significant when present but less so when absent (Muir et al, 1987) (Table 2.2).

A **superficial** burn (Figure 2.1) involves only the surface epithelium. It is characterised by mild pain, erythema (redness), dry skin, slight oedema and a lack of blisters. Skin functions remain intact. The burn will generally heal within 2–3 days and may be accompanied by flaking or peeling. A typical sunburn is an example of this.

A **partial thickness** burn involves the deeper layers of the epidermis or the upper levels of the dermis, and skin functions are lost. In a superficial partial thickness burn (Figure 2.2), the deeper layers of the epidermis are injured, and there is characteristic erythema, blister formation, marked oedema and pain, although the hair follicles, sebaceous glands and sweat glands are spared. Such an

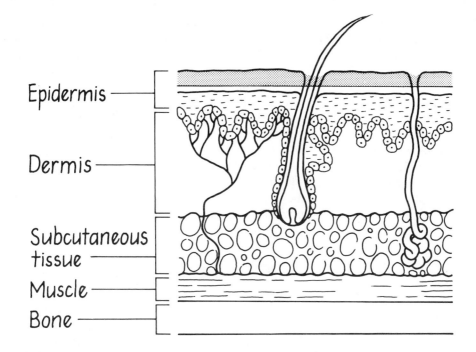

Epidermis

Dermis

Subcutaneous tissue

Muscle

Bone

Fig 2.1 Superficial burn

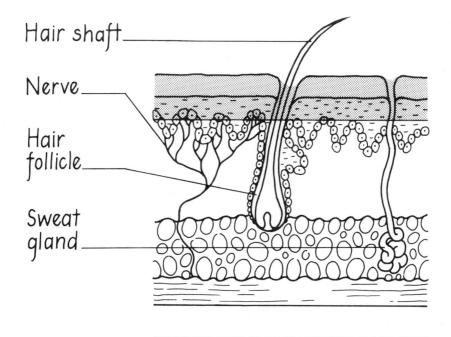

Hair shaft

Nerve

Hair follicle

Sweat gland

Fig 2.2 Partial thickness burn

injury usually heals within 7–10 days, with mild or no scarring. In a **deep partial thickness** burn (Figure 2.3), there is destruction of the epidermis as well as the upper levels of the dermis, and only the deeper parts of the hair follicles or the sweat glands survive. If there is no infection, these burns may heal without grafting in about 3–4 weeks, although scarring may occur.

A **full thickness** burn (Figure 2.4) involves destruction of the epidermis, dermis and epidermal derivatives, and skin functions are lost. Such burns vary in appearance from marble-white to mahogany coloured, to charred, dry wounds. Thrombosed vessels may be visible beneath the injured skin. There is marked oedema, and such a burn is not usually painful to the touch owing to destruction of the nerve endings. Regeneration is slow, and much granulation tissue forms before being covered by epithelium. Even if skin grafting is commenced early, full thickness burns may quickly contract and produce scarring.

EXTENT OF INJURY

When an individual with a thermal injury is first seen, estimation of the area burned is important. The extent of the injury can be estimated by using the Rule of Nines (Wallace, 1951), which indicates, in an easily remembered form, the percentage of total body surface area accounted for by various parts of the body: 9% each for arms and head; 18% each for the legs, front of trunk and back of trunk (Figure 2.5).

In children, these percentages change, since the head and trunk represent a larger proportion of the total body surface area. Therefore, the Lund–Browder chart more accurately determines the extent of the burn (Lund and Browder, 1944) (Figure 2.6). At the Nottingham Burns Unit, a series of body charts have been designed that are more representative of changing body proportion with increasing age (Figure 2.7). Being easier to use, it was found that these charts led to a better estimate by the casualty doctor of the body surface area that had been burned (Wilson et al, 1987). For parts of the body that have only small areas of burn, it is useful to remember that the palmar surface of the patient's hand constitutes about 1% of the body surface area. Areas of erythema should not be included as burned tissue.

A major burn injury is defined as any burn involving greater than 15% total body surface area in an adult, or 10% in a child and these individuals should be transferred to a Burns Unit as soon as possible. Similarly, burns in critical areas, including the hands, face, feet and perineum, are optimally managed at a burn centre. Major inhalation injury, associated trauma and chemical or electrical injuries are also indications for transfer.

CLINICAL HISTORY

The history of the burn injury must be thorough but concise. The time of the incident and type of burning materials must be determined. Some fuels, such as

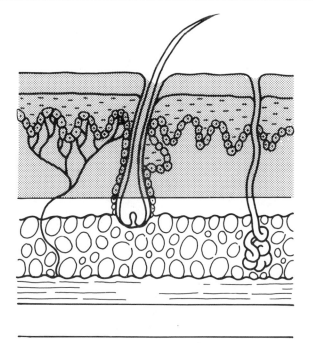

Fig 2.3 Deep partial thickness burn

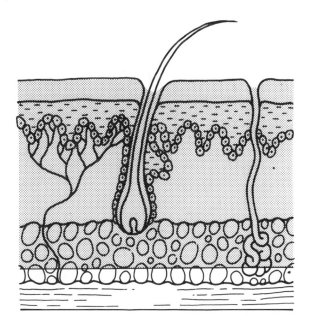

Fig 2.4 Full thickness burn

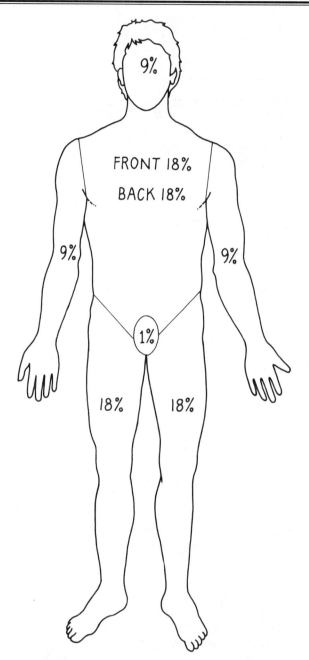

Fig 2.5 Rule of Nines

NAME _____ WARD _____ NUMBER _____ DATE _____

AGE _____ ADMISSION WEIGHT _____

LUND AND BROWDER CHARTS

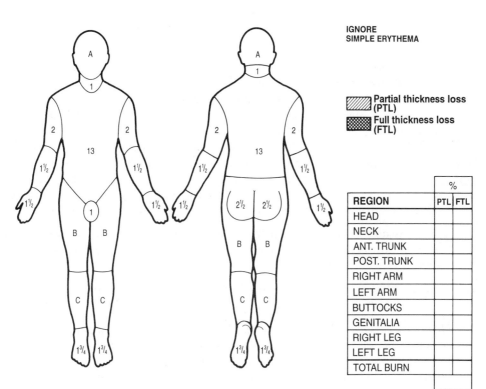

IGNORE
SIMPLE ERYTHEMA

Partial thickness loss (PTL)

Full thickness loss (FTL)

REGION	%	
	PTL	FTL
HEAD		
NECK		
ANT. TRUNK		
POST. TRUNK		
RIGHT ARM		
LEFT ARM		
BUTTOCKS		
GENITALIA		
RIGHT LEG		
LEFT LEG		
TOTAL BURN		

RELATIVE PERCENTAGE OF BODY SURFACE AREA AFFECTED BY GROWTH

AREA	AGE 0	1	5	10	15	ADULT
A = ½ OF HEAD	9½	8½	6½	5½	4½	3½
B = ½ OF ONE THIGH	2¾	3¼	4	4½	4½	4¾
C = ½ OF ONE LEG	2½	2½	2¾	3	3¼	3½

Fig 2.6 Lund and Browder chart

petrol, produce especially severe burns (Williams et al, 1990). Vapours from burning plastics cause a chemical pulmonary injury, especially if the fire has occurred in an enclosed space (Prien and Traber, 1988). The risk of blunt or penetrating injury is increased if there was an explosion and if the individual jumped or fell from a burning building or was burned in a motor vehicle accident.

A history of tobacco use increases the risk of pulmonary complications. A surprising percentage of patients sustain thermal burns as a result of ethanol or drug abuse (Parks et al, 1989). Acute substance withdrawal may complicate fluid resuscitation.

MORTALITY

Survival or death following a burn is highly dependent on the age of the victim and the extent of the injury. Other factors play lesser, although still important roles, and ultimate survival depends on successful management of the patient both initially and through the course of a number of potential complications. Bull (1971) devised a table of statistical values of mortality based on the patient's age and the percentage area of body burned (Table 2.3).

Since Bull's first publication, a number of further studies have identified additional characteristics of burned patients that have significant bearing upon their survival. Although it is universally agreed that age and percentage body surface area burned are two of the most important criteria, there are a variety of factors involved in the burned patient that may also affect the final prognosis:

1. *Age* It is now well established that, for a given size of burn, the prognosis worsens with advancing years after early adult life. There is some controversy over survival rates in early life.

2. *Gender* Most studies have reported mortality as being higher in females (Moores et al, 1975).

3. *Medical history* The pre-existing health of the individual has a crucial bearing on the outcome of the burn injury. A number of factors, including diabetes mellitus, atherosclerosis, chronic renal failure, cirrhosis, collagen vascular disease, steroid use, malignancy, leucopenia secondary to chemotherapeutic agents, and

Table 2.3 Statistical values of mortality with age and percentage area of body burned (Adapted from Bull (1971) and reproduced with kind permission of *The Lancet* Ltd.)

Area of body burned (%)	Age (years)								
	0–4	5–14	15–24	25–34	35–44	45–54	55–64	65–74	75+
93+	1.0	1.0	1.0	1.0	1.0	1.0	1.0	1.0	1.0
83–92	0.9	0.9	0.9	0.9	1.0	1.0	1.0	1.0	1.0
73–82	0.7	0.8	0.8	0.9	0.9	1.0	1.0	1.0	1.0
63–72	0.5	0.6	0.6	0.7	0.8	0.9	1.0	1.0	1.0
53–62	0.3	0.3	0.4	0.5	0.7	0.8	0.9	1.0	1.0
43–52	0.2	0.2	0.2	0.3	0.5	0.6	0.8	1.0	1.0
33–42	0.1	0.1	0.1	0.2	0.3	0.4	0.6	0.9	1.0
23–32	0	0	0	0.1	0.1	0.2	0.4	0.7	1.0
13–22	0	0	0	0	0	0.1	0.2	0.4	0.7
3–12	0	0	0	0	0	0	0.1	0.2	0.4
0–2	0	0	0	0	0	0	0	0.1	0.3

0.1 = 10% mortality; 0.9 = 90% mortality.

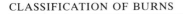

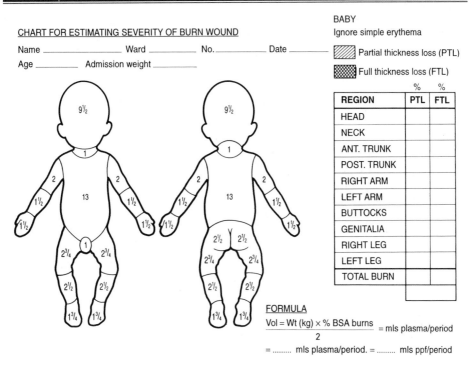

Fig 2.7a   Chart for estimating severity of burn wound for a baby

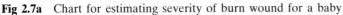

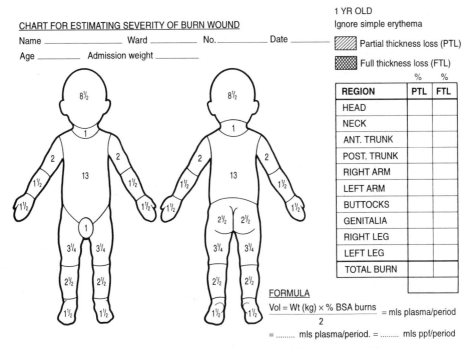

Fig 2.7b   Chart for estimating severity of burn wound for a 1-year-old

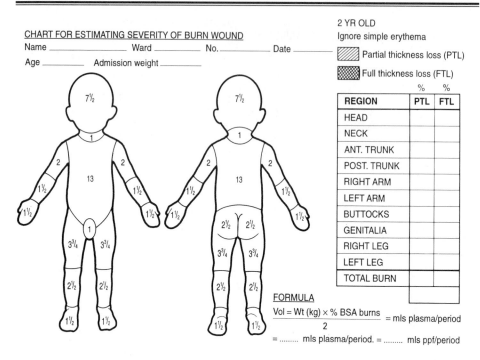

Fig 2.7c   Chart for estimating severity of burn wound for a 2-year-old

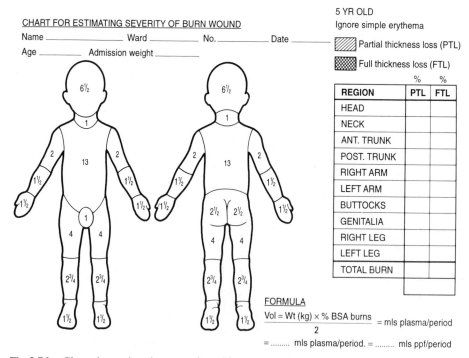

Fig 2.7d   Chart for estimating severity of burn wound for a 5-year-old

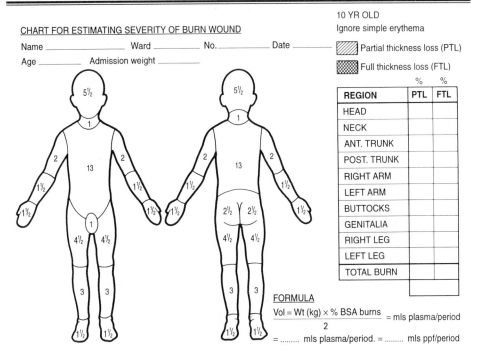

CHART FOR ESTIMATING SEVERITY OF BURN WOUND

10 YR OLD
Ignore simple erythema

Name _____ Ward _____ No._____ Date _____

▨ Partial thickness loss (PTL)

Age _____ Admission weight _____

▩ Full thickness loss (FTL)

REGION	% PTL	% FTL
HEAD		
NECK		
ANT. TRUNK		
POST. TRUNK		
RIGHT ARM		
LEFT ARM		
BUTTOCKS		
GENITALIA		
RIGHT LEG		
LEFT LEG		
TOTAL BURN		

FORMULA

$$\frac{\text{Vol} = \text{Wt (kg)} \times \% \text{ BSA burns}}{2} = \text{mls plasma/period}$$

= .... mls plasma/period. = ... mls ppf/period

Fig 2.7e   Chart for estimating severity of burn wound for a 10-year-old

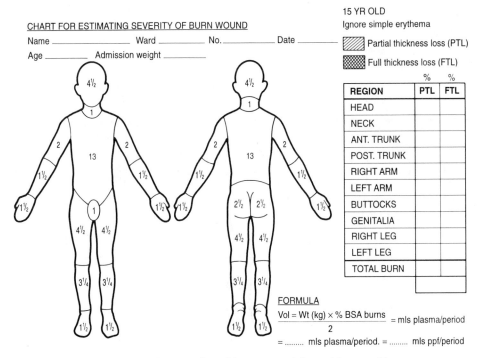

CHART FOR ESTIMATING SEVERITY OF BURN WOUND

15 YR OLD
Ignore simple erythema

Name _____ Ward _____ No._____ Date _____

▨ Partial thickness loss (PTL)

Age _____ Admission weight _____

▩ Full thickness loss (FTL)

REGION	% PTL	% FTL
HEAD		
NECK		
ANT. TRUNK		
POST. TRUNK		
RIGHT ARM		
LEFT ARM		
BUTTOCKS		
GENITALIA		
RIGHT LEG		
LEFT LEG		
TOTAL BURN		

FORMULA

$$\frac{\text{Vol} = \text{Wt (kg)} \times \% \text{ BSA burns}}{2} = \text{mls plasma/period}$$

= .... mls plasma/period. = ... mls ppf/period

Fig 2.7f   Chart for estimating severity of burn wound for a 15-year-old

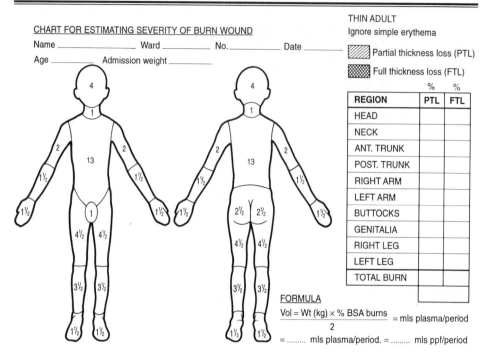

Fig 2.7g   Chart for estimating severity of burn wound for a thin adult

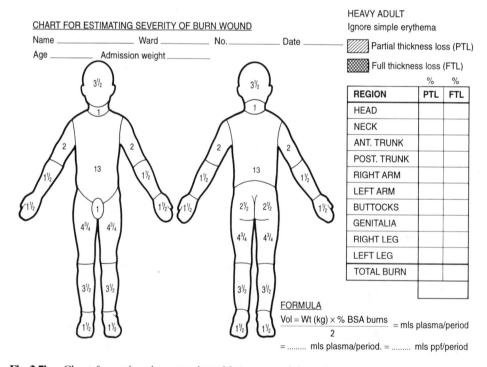

Fig 2.7h   Chart for estimating severity of burn wound for a heavy adult

immunodeficiency states, markedly increase the mortality of thermal injury (Zawacki et al, 1979).

4. *Total body surface area* The percentage of total body surface area burned remains one of the factors most closely associated with mortality. Owing to the increased risk of sepsis, and the demands placed upon the patient by surgery for wound closure, greater nutritional needs and higher blood loss, a deep burn represents a considerably more severe injury in terms of prognosis than does a partial thickness burn of the same area.

5. *Site* The part of the body burned may have some bearing on prognosis, if for instance it is associated with a higher risk of infection or reflects the external injury related to a respiratory burn. Moores et al (1975) found that perineal burns had a significantly higher mortality. Burns to the face may also be associated with a poorer prognosis (Berry et al, 1982).

6. *Type of burn* There is little evidence that the mechanism of burning injury affects subsequent prognosis, providing other factors, such as percentage of deep burn and respiratory injury, are held constant.

7. *Respiratory injury* Inhalation injury or direct thermal damage to the respiratory lining confers a reduced prognosis on the burned patient (Clark et al, 1986). Many of the fatalities in house fires occur as the result of inhalation of hot smoke and other toxic fumes from the conflagration, particularly with the burning of certain foams used for the construction of modern furniture. Deaths from smoke inhalation have increased in recent years and are now the most important single cause of death in burns patients (Muir et al, 1987).

8. *Other injuries* Concomitant injury may markedly influence survival or recovery from the burn injury.

Very few deaths occur purely as a result of the burn itself, most deriving from complications following the injury. Irreversible early shock with renal shut-down still occurs and is the cause of death in about 15% of cases (Curreri et al, 1980). The majority of deaths (60–80%), however, are due to one or more complications. The principal complications are related to the respiratory system, and are either acute, from the injury itself, or delayed, as in pulmonary oedema (Rylah, 1992).

References

Berry CC, Wachtel TL and Frank HA (1982) An analysis of factors which predict mortality in hospitalised burns patients. *Burns* **9:** 38.

Bull JP (1971) Revised analysis of mortality due to burns. *Lancet* **ii:** 1133.

Clark CJ, Reid WH, Gilmour WH and Campbell D (1986) Mortality probability in victims of fire trauma: revised equation to include inhalation injury. *British Medical Journal* **292:** 1303.

Curreri PW, Luterman A, Braun DW et al (1980) Burn injury analysis of survival and hospitalisation time for 937 patients. *Annals of Surgery* **192:** 472.

Dyer C (1988) Burn wound management: an update. *Plastic Surgery Nursing* (spring): 6–12.

Dyer C and Roberts D (1990) Thermal trauma. *Nursing Clinics of North America* **25**(1): 85–117.

Hobbs CJ (1986) When are burns not accidental? *Archives of Disease in Childhood* **61:** 357–361.

Jackson D McG (1953) The diagnosis of the depth of burning. *British Journal of Surgery* **40:** 588.

Kemble JV and Lamb BE (1987) *Practical Burns Management*. London: Hodder & Stoughton.

Lund CC and Browder NC (1944) Estimation of areas of burns. *Surgery, Gynecology and Obstetrics* **79:** 352–358.

Moores B, Rahman MM, Browning FSC and Settle JAD (1975) Discriminant function analysis of 570 consecutive burn patients admitted to the Yorkshire Regional Burns Centre 1966–1973. *Burns* **1:** 135.

Muir IFK, Barclay TL and Settle JAD (1987) *Burns and their Treatment*, 3rd edn. London: Butterworth.

Parks JG, Noguchi TT and Klatt EC (1989) The epidemiology of fatal burn injuries. *Journal of Forensic Science* **34:** 399–406.

Prien T and Traber DL (1988) Toxic smoke compounds and inhalation injury – a review. *Burns* **14:** 451–460.

Purdue GF, Hunt JL and Prescott PR (1988) Child abuse by burning – an index of suspicion. *Journal of Trauma* **28:** 221–224.

Rylah LTA (1992) *Critical Care of the Burned Patient*. Cambridge: Cambridge University Press.

Wallace AB (1951) The exposure treatment of burns. *Lancet* **i:** 501.

Wardrope J and Smith JAR (1992) *The Management of Wounds and Burns*. Oxford: Oxford University Press.

Westaby S (ed.) (1989) *Trauma – Pathogenesis and Treatment*. Oxford: Heinemann Medical.

Williams JB II, Ahrenholz DH, Solem LD et al (1990) Gasoline burns: the preventable cause of thermal injury. *Journal of Burn Care and Rehabilitation* **11:** 446–450.

Wilson GR, Fowler CA and Housden PL (1987) A new burn area assessment chart. *Burns* **13**(5): 401–405.

Zawacki BE, Azen SP, Imbus SH et al (1979) Multifactorial probit analysis of mortality in burned patients. *Annals of Surgery* **189:** 1–5.

3

Nursing Children following Burn Trauma

The thoughtful, knowledgeable, sensitive nursing care that the burn-injured child receives has a profound impact on his survival and quality of life (Trofino, 1991).

This chapter highlights the causes of burn injury in children and the associated risk variables. Non-accidental injury is also mentioned. The complication of burns encephalopathy and toxic shock syndrome are identified, and signs, symptoms and management are discussed. Psychological care and the importance of family-centred care are also outlined.

CAUSES OF BURNS AND SCALDS IN CHILDREN

Seventy per cent of burns occur in children under 5 years of age, the most common age being 1–2 years, and the boy:girl ratio being 3:2. Flame burns can affect children of all ages, whereas contact burns are usually only a problem in the very young. Scalds occur mainly in the under-4 age group, both sexes being equally affected. The boy:girl ratio for serious scalds is approximately 1.3:1.

In 1989 in England and Wales, there were 90 child fatalities resulting from burns, and 5 from scalds. Approximately 5000–6000 children are admitted to hospital per annum (roughly equal numbers with burns and scalds), with an estimated 20 000 outpatient attendances to Accident and Emergency Departments for burns, and 30 000 for scalds (Child Accident Prevention Trust, 1991).

There is a strong link between burning/scalding accidents and low economic status (Child Accident Prevention Trust, 1991). Studies have shown links with poor housing, overcrowding and family stress. Serious burns are noted to be slightly less common in the summer months.

There has been a decrease in the number of deaths from burns, linked to a reduction in clothing fires, because of low-flammability requirements for night-dresses and a move from open fires to central heating and improved fireguards. However, the number of non-fatal burns has changed little over the last 20 years. A downward trend has also been noted in scald fatalities, owing to improved treatment and management. This fall has now levelled out, and a similar trend has been seen in non-fatal accidents.

Tougher laws may be needed to help to reduce the number of burns and scalds still further, for example, in moves such as the recent introduction of a British Standard for fireworks and a successful fireworks education campaign. In this area, cost may also be significant, families opting to attend organised fireworks displays. However, more education is still needed for parents and children.

The *main causes of injury* are:

- Babies and toddlers reaching and grabbing to get near unguarded fires
- Cups within easy reach
- Irons standing on the floor
- Parents holding a baby and hot drink
- Unsupervised baths (parents may be called away to answer the telephone and the toddler climbs in)
- Pulling flexes of kettles that have been left dangling (coiled flexes help to reduce this)
- Overhanging pan handles on the cooker

Among older children, especially boys aged between 9 and 14 years of age, ignorance of the danger of flammable liquids, for example those used to light bonfires, petrol and aerosols sniffed and then followed by smoking, can lead to severe burns.

The *products involved* (not in order of importance) are:

- Matches and smokers' materials
- Bonfires and open coal fires
- Cookers, saucepans and chip pans
- Heaters, such as electric fires
- Cups and mugs containing hot liquids
- Hot fat and oils
- Kettles
- Flammable nightwear
- Toxic fumes from non-combustion, modified foam-filled furniture
- Irons
- Curling tongs
- Live wires
- Baths and showers
- Oven cleaners
- Fireworks
- Motorbikes
- Sunshine

Pearce (1989) carried out a research study in the Nottingham Paediatric Accident and Emergency Department between 1 June 1988 and 30 November 1988, and discovered that most accidents occurred in the afternoon or evening and at meal times.

Hopefully, the future will see a continued reduction in the number of burn and scald injuries with continuing health education.

NON-ACCIDENTAL INJURY

Hobbs (1989) gives the following definitions:

'Accident' – a lapse in usual protection given to the child.

'Neglect' – inadequate or negligent parenting; failing to protect the child.

'Abuse' – deliberately inflicting injury.

About 2% of children who suffer from burns are the victims of non-accidental injury and 10% of all abused children suffer from burns (Jones et al, 1993). All staff working with burn-injured children must be constantly alert for any signs of child abuse, and ensure that immediate and effective action is taken in all suspected cases.

The assessment should be multidisciplinary, involving medical staff, paediatricians, nurses, health visitors and social workers. The 'at risk' register should be checked if there is a suspicion of non-accidental injury and immediately following admission. Both medical and nursing records must be very detailed, relationships and reactions of the family being recorded. Photographs should also be taken on admission, and accurate diagrams drawn.

Neglect, for example a child sustaining a burn or scald on a paralysed limb or after being left unattended in the bath, is much more common than is non-accidental injury. Improbable accidents do occur; in one case, a strange burn to a child's back was the result of a faulty paddling pool melting onto the child in the sun.

The parents and child need a lot of support if a non-accidental injury is suspected, and care must be taken not to show adverse feelings to the person who has abused. It is also very important not to wrongly accuse or judge.

The peak age of children being deliberately burned is during the third year of their life:

- *Scalds* – for example from dipping a child into boiling water, causing scalds to the perineum and genitalia, may be used to punish the child
- *Cigarette burns* – a circular mark is unlikely to be caused by a child brushing passed a lit cigarette (Jones et al, 1993). Additional scars can usually be found on other parts of the body
- *Hands* – the dorsal aspect is affected, whereas in accidents, the palmar surface is usually affected. The hand may be held onto a hot object or in hot water
- *Feet* – burns in a stocking distribution, with no splash marks and a clear demarcation line from dipping into hot water. A contact burn to the sole from an iron, curling tongs, etc may also occur
- *Mouth* – from having hot food forced into the mouth
- *Contact burns* – the injury looks like a brand mark, bearing the shape of the object that caused it. The burn is usually dry and of uniform depth

The history is not usually consistent with the story, although some parents will admit to causing the accident. They may not know how the accident happened or may deny it is a burn or scald, the accident may be unwitnessed, the parents may say that the child did not cry, and the child and parents' story may disagree. Parents may be abusive and hostile to staff, and refuse treatment for their child. Mothers may be withdrawn, depressed and seeking help and may show lack of concern or guilt (Hobbs, 1989). The reaction is usually not what is expected from parents of children with an accidental injury. The abused child may be passive, very withdrawn and not complaining about pain, or very anxious, angry or rebellious. If older children refuse to state the cause of their injury, this may be significant (Hobbs, 1989).

Common factors found in non-accidental injury families (Jones et al, 1993) are:

- A high incidence of personality disorder
- Maternal/paternal deprivation in parental social or family histories
- Rigid parental attitudes to discipline
- A distorted perception of the child
- Ignorance of normal childhood behaviour and development
- Impulsive parental behaviour
- Low tolerance of stress
- Adverse social circumstances
- Poor health
- Low social class
- Younger than average parents
- Frequent changes of home
- Larger than average family size
- An atypical family structure
- Frequent marital upsets
- A high unemployment rate
- A high rate of general criminality

The children, as a general group, have the following characteristics:

- Are more likely to be premature or of low birthweight
- Boys are more at risk than girls until adolescence, after which the trend reverses
- The most serious injuries are on the youngest child
- Are most likely to be illegitimate
- Injuries are reported more in older children.

BURNS ENCEPHALOPATHY

Cerebral oedema is an infrequent but life-threatening complication of a burn or scald in a child. It can occur in a child, generally under 5 years of age, with any percentage of burn or scald, usually 3–4 days after the injury. In Nottingham between 1983 and 1987, there were 11 cases, with a 56% mortality.

A possible cause of burns encephalopathy is cellular overhydration and sodium imbalance. Hence in Nottingham, all children with 5–10% burns or scalds are admitted to the Burns Unit for oral fluid resuscitation. The fluid periods are the same as for intravenous resuscitation 4, 4, 4, 6, 6, 12 hours (See chapter 4). Moyers solution (1.5 g sodium bicarbonate and 4 g sodium chloride in 1 litre of water) is given orally to replace the plasma lost and the amount is calculated by weight × % burn. Other fluids for example milk or Dioralyte are given for maintenance; fruit juice is not given owing to its high potassium content neither is free water. Once the resuscitation phase is over, maintenance fluids continue to be restricted, calculated according to weight for a further five days.

TOXIC SHOCK SYNDROME

It is known that burned children are prone to developing toxic shock syndrome. Once 'shock' has occurred, a 50% mortality rate has been reported (Frame *et al*, 1985).

It is thought the cause may be absorption into the circulation of exotoxin from *Staphylococcus aureus* phage type 1 (McAllister et al, 1993), although blood cultures are usually negative. To prevent a *Staphylococcus aureus* infection, all children who have burns or scalds, however small, are prescribed a 5-day course of oral antibiotics of appropriate dose for their size and weight.

The clinical manifestations of toxic shock syndrome may include pyrexia, so both core and peripheral temperatures should be recorded, a difference of more than 3°C giving a poor prognosis. The temperature difference may also be caused by hypovolaemia; urine output, blood pressure and pulse must, therefore, be monitored hourly. If a child's temperature reaches 38.5°C, the medical staff should be informed and a full bacteriological screen commenced. Blood cultures, swabs from burn wounds, ear, nose and throat, and urine and stool specimens should be obtained. Blood samples are taken for full blood count, urea and electrocytes, and a wire sample is screened for urea, electrocytes and osmolality.

Oral paracetamol and ibuprofen are given as anti-pyretics to help reduce the child's temperature and to maintain comfort. The child may also develop a non-specific rash, vomiting and diarrhoea. Some children develop neutrophilia and disseminating intravascular coagulation. The child's level of consciousness needs to be carefully monitored; it may become impaired due to a convulsion or the need for ventilation. Appropriate treatment should be given to correct the signs and symptoms at each stage of the process. This complication is also discussed further in Chapter 4.

FAMILY-CENTRED CARE

Caring for the parents and the family is an essential part of caring for the child. As well as being upset and anxious, parents may well feel guilty about the cause of their child's injuries. They may blame the person who was with the child at the time of the accident. If one was not there, he or she may take their anger out on the partner, at a time when they need one other's support most of all.

It is important to encourage parents to participate in caring for their child, and to involve them in any decisions regarding their child's care. To make these decisions, they need to be given unbiased and complete information in an appropriate and supportive manner (Campbell, 1993). Participating in the care will help them to overcome feelings of guilt, anger and rejection.

The presence of parents has been shown to be beneficial to children, both physiologically and psychologically. Parents thus need to be made to feel welcome and relaxed, because if they are nervous or uneasy, the child may sense this and become frightened himself (Muller et al, 1992).

In 1959 the Platt report recommended that parents should have unrestricted access to their child in hospital (DoH, 1959). Numerous pieces of research since then have stated the importance of parents staying with the child and participating in care (Campbell et al, 1993). Parents should be made to feel part of the team caring for their child. Parents need comfortable accommodation so that they can unwind and rest, taking regular drinks and meals, and information about the hospital, shops and the local area should be given, so that parents feel as well equipped as possible, both mentally and physically, to help support their child.

Some parents may feel they are unable to participate in the care of their child or be resident with them, and they must be offered support and not made to feel guilty – a single parent with other children at home, and no-one to help, would not find it possible to be resident. Especially in cases such as this, the health-care system needs to be flexible, accessible and responsive to the family's needs; for example, if parents are not resident, but would like to be there when a child's dressings are changed, arrangements should be made to choose a time suitable for all concerned.

It is important to implement appropriate policies and programmes that are comprehensive and provide emotional, spiritual, cultural and financial support to meet the needs of the family. Research by Goulding (1992) has shown that financial difficulties are not well catered for. As Burns Units cover a wide geographical area, cost can be a real problem when a child is in hospital. Multidisciplinary teams would do well to remember that the family is constant in the child's life, while the other teams caring for the child come and go (Campbell et al, 1993).

PSYCHOLOGICAL NEEDS

Children have needs different from those of adults, and these vary according to their age (Kemble and Lamb, 1987). Children need to be cared for in an appropriate environment and by appropriately trained staff.

It is important to learn as much about the children's normal stage of development, what or whom they like and dislike, their hobbies and personality, etc., so that any changes can be detected and routine can be continued as much as possible.

Play is necessary for a child's normal development, and a wide range of toys is needed to cater for all ages. Play can be used to educate children about their care, and as a way for them to express their feelings about the accident and work their way through fears and worries. Play, for example videos, blowing bubbles and imagination, can be used to distract children during procedures. It can also be useful for physiotherapy; a child may not perform standard finger exercises, but will push buttons on a computer or pick up toys. Blowing bubbles can also be used as a breathing exercise. Children need a playroom that is a safe area and free from treatment procedures. A nursery nurse/play specialist fulfils a very important role in a child's stay in hospital.

Explanations to children must be at the appropriate level according to the child's stage of development (Piggett and Tandinhelder, 1969). Children under 2 years of age need someone familiar with them, as they like to explore but have no concept of safety. At all ages, it is important to provide information for parents so that they are able to explain to their child what is happening. Regression can occur at any age to any hospitalised sick child. For example, a toilet-trained toddler may start bed-wetting, or an older child may want his parents around, whereas at home he prefers his friends (Swanick, 1990).

2–6 Years Old

Explanations need to be immediate and related to the present environment. Time can be explained in relation to something familiar to the child, for example meal times. Parents should be encouraged to leave personal items to show that they are returning. In a child's view, illness is caused by external factors, as children are unable to conceive internal illness; they may feel that they are ill because they have been bad and are being punished – reassurance is, therefore, needed to overcome this (Swanick, 1990).

7–11 Years Old

At this age, children can start to apply thinking and reasoning to real objects and events and begin to understand cause and event: they can understand that something external can be caused by internal problems. They can name and draw people, so uncomplicated drawings and explanations can be useful for teaching (Swanick, 1990).

Adolescents

Adolescents understand that illness can be caused by a variety of factors, and that their organs can malfunction, but they may worry unduly as a result of incomplete knowledge of internal processes (Swanick, 1990).

Psychological problems are not immediately resolved on discharge. The child and family have to come to terms with scarring and aftercare, as the damage is visible and permanent. Problems such as nightmares and sleepless nights are usually resolved by 3 months; if they are not, or if there are other problems, the child can be referred to a psychologist for further help and support (Forshaw, 1990). Some families find support by discussing problems at the Outpatients Department when they attend for their appointment, or by meeting other people who have been through a similar experience. Different people find different ways of coping, but support from the Burns Unit should always be available.

It has been found that families from low social economic classes cope better, as there are other, more pressing, problems to deal with (Forshaw, 1990), but the family must never be forgotten, as they may also require psychological help in order to cope with the injury.

SUMMARY

Caring for a child with a burn injury differs from that of an adult due to a variety of factors. These may include different physical responses and needs, decreased cooperation, increased psychological needs and different emotional needs (Kemble and Lamb, 1987). Meeting the needs of the child's parents and family is an essential part of caring for a child and should be considered carefully during the course of hospitalization and following the child's discharge from the Burns Unit. A burn injury is a traumatic experience for any individual irrespective of age. However, in caring for children the burn team needs to acknowledge that the thoughtful, knowledgeable and sensitive care that a child receives following burn injuries has a profound impact on survival and quality of life.

References

Campbell S (1993) Keeping in the family. *Child Health* **1**(1): 17–20.
Campbell S, Kelly P and Summergill P (1993) Putting the family first. *Child Health* **1**(2): 59–60.
Child Accident Prevention Trust (1991) *Burns and Scalds*. Milton Keynes: CAPT.
Department of Health (1959) *The Welfare of Children in Hospital*. Report of the Committee on Child Health Services. (Platt Report). London: HMSO.
Forshaw A (1990) Proven methods. *Paediatric Nursing* **2**(8): 20–21.
Frame JD, Eve MD and Hocked ME (1985) The toxic shock syndrome in burned children. *Burns* **11**: 234.
Goulding J (1992) *The Costs of Visiting Children in Hospital*. London: Action for Sick Children.
Hobbs CJ (1989) ABC of child abuse. *British Medical Journal* **298**: 1304–1308.
Jones DN, Pickett J, Oates MR and Barbor P (1993) *Understanding Child Abuse*. Basingstoke: Macmillan.
Kemble JVH and Lamb B (1987) *Practical Burns Management*. London: Hodder & Stoughton.
McAllister RMR, Mercer NSG, Morgan BDG and Sanders R (1993) Early diagnosis of staphylococcal toxaemia in burned children. *Burns* **19**: 22–25.
Muller DJ, Harris PJ, Wattleys L and Taylor JD (1992) *Nursing Children – Psychology and Research in Practice*, 2nd edn. London: Chapman & Hall.

Pearce S (1989) Researching burns and scalds. *Paediatric Nursing* **1**(10): 13.
Piggett J and Tandinhelder B (1969) *The Psychology of the Child*. London: Routledge & Kegan Paul.
Swanwick M (1990) Knowledge and control. *Paediatric Nursing* **2**(5): 18.
Trofino RB (1991) *Nursing Care of the Burn Injured Patient*. Philadelphia: FA Davis.

4

Management in the

First 48 Hours following

Burn Trauma

An estimated 2 million people are burned each year. Of these, 70 000 require hospitalisation, and 6000–9000 die of their injuries. Until the middle of the 20th century, a massive burn was universally fatal, death being due to 'burns toxaemia'. It is only in the past 50 years that the pathophysiology of burns 'shock' has been appreciated and appropriate treatment regimens established. The chances of surviving massive burns are today much improved, but without appropriate treatment, the outlook is no better than at the turn of the century.

This chapter outlines the management necessary in the first 48 hours after injury, including the initial assessment and history-taking. Fluid and electrolyte management will be discussed, as will the systemic effects on the patient, and methods of monitoring and minimising potential complications during the resuscitation phase.

Although much of the treatment starts, and complications may arise, in the first 48 hours, there is no natural break in the clinical situation. Treatment continues until the wound is closed and beyond, and complications can occur anywhere along the way.

FIRST AID

Should you be unlucky enough to be the first person at the scene of a burn injury, the initial step is to prevent further injury to the casualty. This may simply mean removing him from the source of the heat or extinguishing burning clothes. Clothing soaked in hot fluid acts like a hot poultice, and should therefore be removed or cooled with cold water. Cooling in other circumstances is of debatable value, and although it may soothe the burn, it may also induce hypothermia. However, prompt application of cold water to a burn eases pain (Davies, 1982) and according to Lawrence (1986) quenches residual heat thus reducing tissue damage caused by the burning or scalding agent. The current first aid treatment recommended for burns and scalds by the British Burn Association is prompt cooling of the burn area with copious amounts of tap water for 10–20 mins (Lawrence, 1987; Lawrence, 1996). The application of a temporary dressing e.g. cling film may then be applied to the burn wound (Wilson and French, 1987) if appropriate, in preparation for transfer of the individual to the Accident and Emergency Department. However, initiating these measures should certainly not delay the transport of the patient to hospital.

THE ACCIDENT AND EMERGENCY DEPARTMENT

As with any other trauma patient, initial management in the Accident and Emergency Department should be interlinked with the guidelines laid down by advanced trauma and life support (ATLS) courses.

1. *Airway* Ensure that the patient has a patent airway and no breathing difficulties. Severe facial burns and/or a history of inhalation injury should raise the question of ventilatory support, and an anaesthetic review should be requested. Oxygen by facemask can be applied as an interim measure.

2. *Circulation* The circulatory state should be checked by pulse and blood pressure readings, and signs of shock should be elicited.

3. *History* A brief history of the events, including the time and nature of the accident, should be obtained.

4. *Examination* A brief general examination should be performed, assessing the conscious state, the presence of other injuries or illnesses and the extent of the burn injury. From this, the need for admission and/or intravenous fluids can be obtained. Children with a burn of 10% or more body surface area and adults with a burn of 15% or more, require intravenous fluids, but smaller burns may need admission because of their site or severity.

5. *Intravenous access* If intravenous fluids are required, good access is essential. Large-bore peripheral cannulae, which can be inserted through burnt skin if necessary, are preferable. Cut-downs onto large veins may be necessary if the patient is peripherally shut down, but central vein cannulation is best avoided if possible. Fluid infusion may then be commenced with either plasma or a suitable plasma expander.

6. *Blood samples* These can often be taken at the same time as the intravenous access is being established. Urea and electrolyte levels, a full blood count and a haematocrit should be requested. In large burn injuries, the patient should also be blood grouped, and if there is a possibility of an inhalation injury, carboxy-haemoglobin levels should also be measured.

7. *Analgesia* Intravenous opiates are the analgesics of choice, as they can be titrated against the patient's pain. Oral or intramuscular drugs will have erratic absorption during the 'shock' phase and will give poor pain control. Inhalational agents such as entonox may also be helpful.

8. *Catheterisation* If the burn area is over 10% of body surface area in children, over 15% in adults or involves the perineum, the passage of a urinary catheter should be considered. The volume of urine drained at this time should also be measured.

9. *The individual's general condition* should be reassessed, looking for any change in the general state of the patient and ensuring that the airway is still patent and the infusions running. Other injuries should also be reassessed.

10. *The burn* should be reassessed, using the Lund and Browder (1944) chart or the Nottingham percentage by age charts (Wilson et al, 1987) to determine its size, and an attempt should be made to differentiate partial and full thickness burns. The need for escharotomies should also be evaluated when circumferential burns are evident on the limbs, neck or trunk.

11. *Dressings* If the patient is to be transferred to a Burns Unit, a temporary dressing should be applied. This should ideally be easy to apply and remove, painless on removal, non-stick, sterile and waterproof. 'Cling-film', as advocated by Wilson and French (1987), fulfils most of these criteria and is also very cheap. If the patient is to be discharged, a definitive dressing should be applied.

12. *Transfer* should be arranged if required, but only once the above measures have been taken and the patient is fit for transfer. The Burns Unit is often some distance away, so the patient's condition should be stable and all intravenous lines carefully secured for the journey. If the patient is intubated, an anaesthetist will have to accompany him.

THE BURNS UNIT

The immediate aspects of management should all have been commenced in the Accident and Emergency Department (unless the patient is admitted directly) and need to be continued by the Burns team. First priority is checking:

- The airway
- That the intravenous infusion is running
- The urinary catheter
- Analgesia
- Blood samples
- The patient's weight

If any of these aspects have not yet been addressed, now is the time to do it. Once this has been completed, a more detailed history and examination can be performed, and the fluid requirements calculated.

History

Probably the first step in treating any trauma patient is to establish the history of the event. The treatment of the burns patient is no different.

The main points to establish are the time of the accident (as all the resuscitation formulae start from this point, rather than the time the patient is first seen) and the causal agents. These may be roughly divided into four groups: wet, dry, chemical and electrical. Knowing the causal agent will often help in estimating the severity of the burn.

1.   Wet burns are generally scald injuries from hot fluids or steam, and account for a large proportion of burn injuries, especially in children under 5 years.

2.   Dry burns occur from flame or hot objects, from either direct contact or radiated heat, and are more common in adults.

3.   Chemical burns arise from a variety of substances, usually acid or alkali, which may continue to burn long after the initial exposure. The severity of the injury depends on the strength of the chemical involved, the duration of exposure and any first aid that was given. The main treatment for most chemicals is removal of the agent by copious irrigation, but some have specific treatments, for example phosphorus burns, and hydrofluoric acid burns. If there is any doubt about the type of chemical involved, specialist advice should be sought from the manufacturer or from Guy's Hospital Poisons Unit, London.

4.   Electrical injuries may have an element of thermal damage, either from direct contact or from a flash injury, as well as an electrocution injury. Where an electrocution injury is suspected, entry and exit wounds should be sought and an ECG performed to check for arrhythmias. It is generally accepted that these patients should be admitted for 24-hour cardiac monitoring, although this is debatable if the ECG is normal.

Not only is the type of burn important, but also the length of exposure will determine the severity. A flash of intense heat may only produce erythema or superficial damage, whereas prolonged exposure to relatively low heat can still cause full thickness damage. Removal of clothing soaked in hot liquid is important in this respect, as it may retain heat and thus increase the depth of the burn.

Having established the nature and timing of the burn, it is important to establish the circumstances of the accident. Fires in enclosed spaces carry a significant risk of inhalation injury. Accidents at work may be open to negligence claims if safety measures were not enforced. There may also be predisposing factors, either at the place of the accident or in the patient himself, for example epilepsy and diabetes. Not all burn injuries are accidental, and this applies equally to adults as well as children. In adults, self-harm and assault victims form a significant number of admissions, and it may be necessary to involve other agencies, such as psychiatrists or the police, in these cases.

Non-accidental injury (NAI) in children should always be suspected where the injury and history do not tally. A past history of injury and signs of old injuries, such as bruising, healed burns, etc., should also raise suspicion. If there is any doubt, the child should be admitted while the Social Services are alerted, the 'at risk' register checked, and review by a paediatrician arranged. Any injuries found should also be photographed at this stage for future reference. If at all possible, all of this should be done without arousing the suspicions of the parents, who can be unnecessarily distressed by unfounded claims of NAI when already feeling guilt over the accident.

As with any other trauma patient, we should not be tempted to concentrate only on the obvious problem. It is all too easy to miss other injuries or medical conditions unless they are specifically elicited. These may pre-date the accident or have occurred at the same time, often playing a role in the cause of the injury; examples are fractures sustained while escaping from a fire and the elderly patient who collapses with a myocardial infarction or cerebrovascular accident while cooking. These other conditions may be more serious than the burn injury, which may well take secondary importance, and treatment should be tailored appropriately.

A full history of the patient's past medical problems is also relevant, as this may well influence subsequent treatment. Any medications taken should be fully documented, along with any allergies and the tetanus status (because if the patient is not covered, immunisation is required).

Assessment

The initial assessment of the burn injury is performed in the Accident and Emergency Department and is mainly a form of triage. Burns of over 10% of total body surface area in children and 15% in adults require admission for intravenous resuscitation. However, smaller burns may require admission because of the site or nature of the burn. Burns of the face often necessitate admission as they swell considerably, making management as an outpatient impractical. Similarly, burns involving the hands, feet or genitalia may represent a small physical area but a difficult management problem.

Assessment of the burn injury involves assessment of both the depth and the body surface area of the burn. Depth may be classified as erythema, superficial, partial thickness, deep partial thickness or full thickness, as described in Chapter 2. In some countries, degrees of burn are used, but this can be confusing as definitions vary. Estimating depth takes into account the appearance of the burn, capillary return and sensation. Erythema is generally ignored as it does not require treatment and does not affect the fluid losses.

Superficial burns are red with a dry bloated appearance and are painful. Partial thickness burns are often blistered, painful and pink, with a good capillary return. Deep partial thickness burns may be blistered, have a deeper red or mottled appearance that does not readily blanch, and may have reduced sensation. Full thickness burns are pain-free and feel tough and leathery, with no capillary function at all.

Various methods have been described for assessing the body surface area of the burn injury, and, as several studies have shown, the area is often miscalculated by as much as 60% or more. The simplest guide to area is to use the patient's hand, which, with the fingers, represents 1% of the body surface. This is useful when estimating small areas, but it is not practical when dealing with large ones.

The Rule of Nines was advocated by Wallace in 1951 (Kyle and Wallace, 1951), and is accurate enough for most practical purposes, as well as being easy to remember. The body is essentially divided into parts that represent 9%, or multi-ples thereof, of the total body surface area, leaving 1% for the genitalia (see Figure 2.5).

More accurate estimations can be gained by using the Lund and Browder charts (Lund and Browder, 1944) available in most Accident and Emergency Departments (see Figure 2.6) or the Nottingham charts (Wilson et al, 1987) (see Figure 2.7). Both rely on accurate drawing of the burn area onto a chart, the areas then being added up. The latter charts are more accurate, as they come in a range from baby to adult sizing, adjusted for the changing ratios of head to body and limbs.

Not only should the depth and area of the burn be assessed, but the site of the burn may well also be relevant to the admission. Burns of certain areas, such as the hands, feet, face and genitalia, require specific treatment, as detailed in Chapter 5. Involvement of the eyes may require a specialist opinion, and fluorescein staining to exclude corneal damage should be carried out early before the lids swell. Where there have been extensive or deep burns of the eyelids, temporary tarsorrhaphy and/or early skin grafting may be necessary to prevent exposure of the cornea.

Where there are circumferential full thickness burns on a limb or the trunk, escharotomies may be needed. Areas of full thickness loss, where tissue elasticity has been lost, will not stretch as the tissues swell following the injury. Where this is circumferential, it will lead to a tourniquet effect, raising tissue pressure and reducing blood flow distally. This may then lead to necrosis and loss of the distal part. Where the burns affect the chest, they may interfere with ventilation.

To allow the areas to swell without these problems requires release of the burn area by splitting the burned tissue down to normal tissues, a technique known as escharotomy. As the burned tissue is anaesthetic, no analgesia is required. The incision should be made through the burned skin along the entire length, down to healthy tissues and avoiding major cutaneous and digital nerves. The patient will often gain considerable relief from this process, as ischaemic tissues are extremely painful.

Evidence of inhalation injury should again be assessed, especially if there are facial burns. Singeing of nasal hairs, soot in the mouth or throat, hoarseness and stridor are all significant signs and indications for intubation. The marked swelling of the face and neck following injury may in itself lead to airway obstruction and be an indication for early intubation. If there is any doubt, the anaesthetist's opinion should be sought earlier rather than later. Inhalational injuries are dealt with in more detail in Chapter 6.

Having fully assessed the burn wound itself, a full medical examination of the patient should be made, looking for any associated illnesses, as outlined earlier.

Fluid Requirements

Fluid loss occurs both from the burn surface, as exudate and blister fluid, and into the surrounding tissues, as oedema. This loss is mainly of plasma and is greatest over the first 8 hours following injury, but it continues until the capillaries recover, after about 36 hours. Overall, these losses can be predicted fairly accurately, and this forms the basis of the various fluid replacement regimens.

Fluid loss as the cause of 'burns shock', rather than toxins released from the burned tissue, was first proposed by Underhill et al (1923), but it was not until 20 years later that this theory was widely accepted. Various formulae were subsequently described to calculate the volumes of fluid replacement necessary (Figure 4.1) (Harkins et al, 1942; Cope and Moore, 1947; Baxter, 1981). Evans et al (1952) produced the first widely publicised formula, relating fluid requirement to the size of the burn and the size of the patient. Equal parts of plasma and saline were used, giving two thirds of the total in the first 24 hours, and the remaining third in the second 24. The Brooke formula (Reiss et al, 1953) gives 3 ml/kg per % BSA burn, but uses less plasma and an increased rate of infusion. This trend continued in America with Moyer in 1965 (Moyer et al, 1965) and Baxter in 1968 (Baxter and Shires, 1968). This formula used 4 ml/kg per % BSA burn of Ringer's lactate in the first 24 hours with no colloid at all, giving half of this in the first 8 hours and half over the next 16 hours. In the UK, Muir and Barclay (1962) continued to use plasma in the Mount Vernon formula, which is still widely used in most units in the UK today:

$$\text{Volume/period} = \frac{\text{Total percentage area of burn} \times \text{weight (kg)}}{2}$$

The first 36 hours is divided into periods of 4, 4, 4, 6, 6 and 12 hours, and the calculated volume is infused in each period, starting from the time of the injury, rather than the time the infusion started (Figure 4.2).

There is still debate over the best fluids to use and the best formula (Demling, 1987). In general, there are three schools of thought: (a) protein should be given from the start along with crystalloid; (b) protein should not be given in the first 24 hours as it is no more effective than is salt water during this time; and (c) a protein infusion should be started at between 8 and 12 hours, using crystalloid or non-protein colloid in the first 8–12 hours as most of the fluid shifts occur during this time (Moncrief, 1972). In general, during the first 48 hours, the patient needs about 0.5 mmol Na/kg per % BSA burn and 2–4 ml fluid/kg per % BSA burn, at least half of which is given in the first 12 hours (Settle, 1982).

In America, crystalloids are mostly used, while in the UK it is mainly colloids in the form of albumin solutions, Human Albumin Solution (HAS) or Human Plasma Protein Fraction (HPPF). Both methods are equally successful, but there is less oedema with colloids and thus fewer complications from ulcers, paralytic ileus and pulmonary problems. However, colloids are expensive and carry the theoretical risk of all blood products, although HAS is heat treated to destroy infective particles.

All the formulae are only guidelines and a point from which to start. Frequent reassessment and adjustment is required for an uneventful resuscitation. At any time during the resuscitation period, the plasma deficit can be calculated from the following formula:

$$\text{Plasma deficit} = \text{blood volume} - \left[\text{blood volume} \times \frac{\text{normal haematocrit}}{\text{observed haematocrit}} \right]$$

Blood volume (ml) being approximately 70 × weight (kg) for adults, and 80 × weight (kg) for children.

Thus, if at any stage, the calculated fluid volumes do not seem to be adequate, the plasma deficit can be calculated and this amount added to the fluids being given, to correct the deficit.

Brooke	• Day 1 – colloid 0.5 ml/kg per % + crystalloid 1.5 ml/kg per % – half in the first 8 hours, half in the next 16 hours • Day 2 – colloid 0.25 ml/kg per % + crystalloid 0.5 ml/kg per % • Maintenance – 5% dextrose 200 ml/m²
Modified Brooke	No colloid. No maintenance • Day 1 – 2 ml/kg per % for adults, or 3 ml/kg per % for children – half in the first 8 hours, half in the next 16 hours • Day 2 – coloid 0.3–0.5 ml/kg per %. No crystalloid
Parkland	• Day 1 – Ringer's lactate 4 ml/kg per %. No colloid or maintenance – half in the first 8 hours, half in the next 16 hours • Day 2 – 700–2000 m colloid to maintain urine output • No crystalloid and 5% dextrose maintenance fluids
Evans	• Day 1 – colloid 1 ml/kg per % + Ringer's lactate 1 ml/kg per % – half in the first 8 hours, half in the next 16 hours – plus 5% dextrose 2000 ml/m² • Day 2 – colloid 0.5 ml/kg per % + Ringer's lactate 0.5 ml/kg per %
Bull and Jackson	• Day 1 – 1–1.5l/10% plasma – half in the first 8 hours, half in the next 16 hours • Day 2 – half this volume over 24 hours • Children – one plasma volume/15% given as above
Sorensen	• Dextran 70 120 ml/% in adults – Half in the first 8 hours, one-quarter in the next 16 hours and in the next 24 hours – Plus 5% dextrose 50 ml/kg maintenance
Monafo	• 250 mEq sodium, 150 mEq lactate, 100 mEq chloride titrated to urine flow, plus liberal 'free water' by mouth (Monafo, 1970)

Fig 4.1 Burn formulae

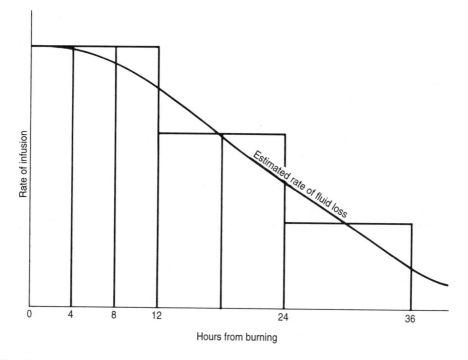

Fig 4.2 Estimated rate of fluid loss

Maintenance Fluids

As well as to compensate for fluid losses from the burn wound, the patient needs fluids for the normal metabolic requirement. This requirement is related to extra renal and evaporative losses, and is increased if the wound is exposed or the patient pyrexial. In the first 24 hours, there will be antidiuretic hormone secretion as part of the 'stress response', and it may be wise to restrict water intake during this time to about 100 ml/hour for adults (starting at about 60 ml/hour and increasing to 100 ml/hour if there are no problems) (Baxter, 1974); children's needs will be considered below.

Burns of more than 25% of total body surface area are usually accompanied by some degree of paralytic ileus, so that absorption from the gut is greatly reduced, and vomiting often occurs. It may be better to keep these patients nil by mouth initially until normal gut function is restored. However, in many units, a policy of early feeding is being advocated; this will be discussed further in Chapter 9. In burns greater than 20% of surface area, it is advisable to pass a nasogastric tube and to aspirate hourly.

Patients with burns of between 10% and 15% of total body surface area should be able to tolerate fluids orally, but if there is vomiting, the maintenance fluid should be given intravenously. Sodium-free solutions should be avoided, especially in children, as there is a significant risk of hyponatraemia and water intoxication

(Batchelor et al, 1961). This leads to cellular overhydration, which may play a role in burns encephalopathy, where there is cerebral irritability, increased temperature, vomiting, fits and eventual coma. In children, it is thus best to use salt-containing solutions such as Dioralyte or milk for maintenance fluids, and avoid salt-free solutions such as fruit juice/squash (Carvajal, 1980).

Maintenance requirements for children are:

- < 10 kg   100 ml/kg per hour
- 10–15 kg   90 ml/kg per hour
- 15–20 kg   80 ml/kg per hour
- 20–25 kg   70 ml/kg per hour
- 25–30 kg   60 ml/kg per hour

If intravenous resuscitation is also in progress, this maintenance volume should be reduced to 75% of the total (100% during oral resuscitation), and this maintenance fluid restriction should continue for the first 5 days post-burn.

Oral Resuscitation

In burns of less than 10% of surface area in children and 15% in adults, oral resuscitation is usually adequate. However, unless the burn is trivial, input and output should still be monitored, and, if the burn is near the critical level, the patient should be regularly reassessed. Also, some areas such as the face lose fluid volumes out of proportion to the size of the burn.

Hypotonic solutions are better tolerated than are isotonic solutions by mouth, and are thus used for this group of patients. Moyer's solution of 3 g salt + 1.5 g sodium bicarbonate per litre (½ teaspoon salt + ½ teaspoon bicarbonate in 2 pints) is a suitable solution (Moyer, 1953), and can be flavoured to make it more palatable.

In children with burns of between 5% and 10% of body surface area, the fluid requirement is calculated by weight × % burn and given as oral Moyer's solution over the same time periods (4, 4, 4, 6, 6, 12 hours) from the time of injury. Maintenance fluid is then given as milk or Dioralyte.

Requirement for Blood

Muir (1961) showed the relationship between red cell destruction and the extent of the full thickness burn. Some cells are actually destroyed by the heat of the burn, and, if this happens in significant numbers, this will be manifest by haemoglobinuria. Others are rendered fragile, so that they are removed from the circulation during the next few hours. However, even in burns of more than 50% of surface area, this loss does not exceed 10% of the total red cell volume. During the main part of the shock phase, further loss continues, for reasons that are not entirely clear.

In general, where there is a large area of full thickness burn, there will be a significant fall in haemoglobin concentration, and the patient will require

transfusion. Where the area of full thickness loss exceeds 10%, the blood requirement is 1% of the patient's normal blood volume for each 1% of full thickness
burn. For an adult, this works out at about one unit of blood for every 10% of
full thickness burn over and above 10% BSA burn. This is usually given in the
sixth period of resuscitation (24–36 hours post injury) so that it does not interfere with the monitoring during the early stages.

Monitoring

Monitoring of the burns patient is mainly aimed at detecting the signs of shock
so that it can be treated appropriately to avoid more serious complications
(Demling, 1987).

1.   *Restlessness* is often a sign of oligaemia and is especially useful in children,
although it may have other causes.

2.   *Skin colour* is also of use. Pink skin indicates dilated arterioles and an adequate
circulation, whereas pallor indicates constricted arterioles. A bluish tinge indicates
stagnation of blood in capillaries that are dilated, and is a bad sign in the severely
shocked patient.

3.   *Pulse and blood pressure* are routinely recorded. Many factors affect the pulse
rate, so that trends in the rate are more important than are hourly fluctuations.
A fall in the blood pressure is a late sign, and monitoring of blood pressure is of
less value than other parameters.

4.   *Skin and deep body temperature* can be recorded, a difference between the
two revealing a degree of vasoconstriction. As the patient's condition improves,
the gap narrows (normally to 1–4°C). The skin temperature is relatively easy to
measure, while the core temperature is measured either rectally or using probes
attached to the catheter or in the external auditory meatus.

5.   *Urine output* reflects the perfusion of the kidney and is thus a useful measurement. However, in the early stages, the output will be affected by, for example,
ADH, catecholamines and angiotensin, which are secreted as part of the 'stress
response'. Thus, there may be wide variation in hourly volumes, so it is important to note the concentration as well to make sense of the readings. ADH is
present for the first 24 hours after injury, so the urine is more concentrated than
the filtrate, and the osmolarity of the urine will be 2–3 times higher than that of
plasma (approximately 300 mOsmol/l). An adequate flow is 0.5–1.0 ml/hour per
kg body weight. Low flow with concentrated urine indicates inadequate resuscitation, whereas reduced concentration and a high flow indicates overtransfusion
(Settle, 1974).

6.   *The haematocrit* is a measure of the proportion of red cells to plasma volume
expressed as either a percentage or a fraction. A raised haematocrit almost always
indicates a low plasma volume, but a normal or low reading does not necessarily
mean adequate resuscitation (as other factors, such as anaemia, may play a role).

Again, absolute values are less relevant than the trend over several readings. Measurements can be made from a skin prick and collecting the blood in a capillary tube, which is then centrifuged. The haematocrit can then be measured directly.

7. *Central venous pressure* (CVP) readings are used extensively in the treatment of major trauma, where there are rapid changes in the haemodynamic state of the patient. In burns shock, the changes are more gradual, so this type of invasive monitoring is seldom necessary. There is also the risk of infection in the burn patient, in addition to other risks from placement of the cannula. Where this type of monitoring is needed, pulmonary artery pressure is probably a better guide than CVP is but it requires the placement of a Swan–Ganz catheter.

8. *Gut absorption* is affected by the circulatory state, and burns of 20% total body surface area or above are more generally accompanied by a paralytic ileus. This may present as vomiting or large amounts of aspirate if a nasogastric tube has been passed. Once adequate resuscitation is underway, gut function will return, and many people advocate early feeding to reduce the risk of bacterial translocation and subsequent sepsis.

Analgesia

Adequate analgesia is essential in the treatment of burns and is dealt with more fully in Chapter 7. As most people know, even a small burn can be excruciatingly painful, but where the burn is deep, it will be relatively pain-free. In the initial stages of treatment, an analgesic is required that gives good pain control, is easily adjustable and has some sedative effects. Oral and intramuscular drugs will have an erratic absorption during the resuscitation period, so the intravenous route is the route of choice. An ideal method of pain control is diamorphine infusion, which can be titrated against the patient's symptoms and increased or reduced as necessary.

Entonox is a useful adjuvant, and can be used in both adults and children by self-administration.

Dressing the burn wound reduces much of the discomfort from the injury and it is often quite soothing once the dressings are in place. The types of dressing used and their management are discussed elsewhere.

COMPLICATIONS

Complications can arise at any stage in the treatment of the burn patient, and may loosely be divided into early and late complications. At this stage, we will deal mainly with those complications arising in the first few days after injury. **However, many of the problems occurring later have their roots in the early management of the patient.**

Renal Failure

Renal failure is largely preventable with adequate resuscitation, and acute tubular necrosis due to hypovolaemia should rarely be seen. However, patients with a burn of 20% or more of total body surface area often have a degree of renal impairment, owing to mixed tubular and glomerular damage, which manifests itself as proteinuria in the first few days after injury. The severity of the damage varies from minor with no adverse effects, to severe with acute oligaemic renal failure, in which there is low flow, fixed osmolarity, low urinary urea:blood urea ratio, low urinary creatinine and rising blood creatinine and urea.

Occasionally, high output renal failure occurs, which is harder to detect as there is a good flow of urine. However, the blood urea rises, with a urine concentration of 350–400 mOsmol/l, and a urinary:blood urea ratio of less than 10.

Treatment of renal failure in the burns patient can be complicated and often requires CVP monitoring to assess the fluid balance, as urinary output cannot be used for this. Overtransfusion is relatively easy to accomplish, and can lead to pulmonary oedema unless there is careful monitoring. In non-oliguric failure, it may be possible to promote a diuresis with osmotic diuretics, but if this fails, dialysis will be necessary. Haemodialysis, peritoneal dialysis or haemofiltration may be used, depending on the patient's condition and the skills available.

Respiratory Complications

Respiratory complications in the early stages of care may arise from inhalational burns and the toxic products of combustion or respiratory distress syndrome may develop later. These problems will be dealt with in greater depth in Chapter 6.

Electrolyte Balance

Electrolyte disturbances are not uncommon in the burns patient during the first few days and, with the volumes of fluid transfused over this time, not entirely unexpected (Baxter, 1974). The main emphasis at this time should be on maintaining adequate volume replacement, as once the patient is taking a normal diet, and providing his renal function is normal, any imbalance will soon be corrected. In some patients, however, there is an abnormality of the cell membranes that allows potassium to leak out and sodium to leak in in abnormal quantities – the so-called 'sick-cell syndrome' – in which the patients become restless and disorientated and overbreathe. This may be difficult to detect, as plasma levels of electrolytes are often normal, but the sodium:potassium ratio in the urine may be reversed. The first step in treatment is to correct any cause of tissue hypoxia, such as unrecognised anaemia, and the administration of glucose and insulin has been shown to be beneficial.

Infection

Infection is a serious problem and in large burns may lead to overwhelming sepsis. The burn wound is a large open area rich in nutrients and devoid of bodily defences in the eschar, which makes it ideal for colonisation once contamination has occurred. Infection only occurs when there are enough organisms present to invade healthy tissue, and will lead to sepsis and septicaemia.

In large burns, there is a degree of immunosuppression with a temporary failure of the local cellular defences, leading to reduced phagocytosis and clearance by the reticulo-endothelial system and impaired response to antigens. The loss of immunoglobulins is transient, but lymphocyte and T-cell activity is reduced by substances released by damaged tissue and bacteria, which allow organisms such as *Staphylococcus aureus*, haemolytic *Streptococcus*, *Pseudomonas* and Acinetobacter to thrive.

The main way to avoid these problems is prevention, using aseptic techniques at all stages. The burn wound is initially sterile, and the aim should be to keep it that way. Dressings should be performed in a clean environment, with gloves and gowns being worn; dead tissue is removed and the wound irrigated before the dressings are applied. Ideally, single cubicles with positive pressure ventilation should be used, with care in hand-washing, etc. to prevent contamination. The use of prophylactic antibiotics is not generally recommended as this encourages the emergence of resistant strains of bacteria, but flucloxacillin is often used in children to prevent staphylococcal colonisation and the potential development of toxic shock syndrome. Early surgery, with the removal of the eschar and skin grafting before colonisation occurs, is a good ideal, but is not always possible to achieve.

The maintenance of adequate nutrition is essential, as is regular bacterial surveillance, wound swabs being taken at every dressing change. The treatment of established infection involves the use of topical and systemic antibiotics, and surgical excision of the eschar.

Gastrointestinal Ulceration

Gastric and duodenal ulceration has been described in burn patients and can lead to serious complications. Superficial erosions are common in the first few days, and may be related to vasoconstriction with reduced mucosal blood flow in the shock phase. True duodenal ulceration (Curling's ulcer) usually develops 10–14 days post-burn. Treatment is again aimed at prevention, with the use of sucralfate (a coating agent), H_2 antagonists, for example cimetidine and ranitidine, and early feeding regimes.

Red Cell Destruction

Red cell destruction occurs to some degree in all deep burns but seldom leads to a loss of more than 10% of red cells. In some cases, there is a rapidly increasing loss owing to increased red cell fragility, which shows as a failure to respond to treatment despite a falling haematocrit. There will also be haemoglobinuria occurring after 12 hours, either for the first time or after a period of clear urine. Treatment is to replace the losses, which may mean massive transfusion.

Glycosuria

Glycosuria is not uncommon and is usually transient, lasting about 48 hours, and with no associated ketonuria. There may be exacerbation of pre-existing diabetes, with glycosuria, ketonuria and raised blood sugar levels, which should be treated symptomatically.

Occasionally, gross hyperglycaemia and glycosuria develop several days after the injury, as a result of adrenal cortical overactivity. This pseudo-diabetes of burns is insulin resistant, and treatment is supportive, with high calorie intake to reduce the muscle wasting until normality returns.

Liver and Pancreas

Liver failure, liver necrosis and pancreatitis have all been described in severe burns, and are probably due to oligaemic problems and subsequent ischaemia.

Toxic Shock Syndrome

Toxic shock syndrome has been described in burnt children and is not related to the burn size (Frame et al, 1985). It is due to toxins released by a specific phage type of *Staphylococcus aureus* that colonises the burn wound. Adults are rarely affected, as they have usually been exposed to the toxin and have the appropriate antibodies. The syndrome develops very rapidly, from the first signs of pyrexia, rash, diarrhoea and vomiting, to complete circulatory collapse and death. There is also a falling platelet and white cell count, although blood cultures are negative. Treatment is the administration of fresh frozen plasma (which contains antibodies) and supportive measures until the child recovers. Treatment should be started early if the condition is suspected as the progression is very rapid.

Burns Encephalopathy

Burns encephalopathy has also been described in burned children and again may develop rapidly. It is thought to result from cellular overhydration and hyponatraemia following the administration of excess salt-poor fluids during the resuscitation period. This can lead to cerebral oedema, with reduced levels of consciousness and fitting. For this reason, the use of water or salt-free solutions is not recommended when treating burned children.

METABOLIC EFFECTS OF BURNS

After any serious injury, including burns, there is a change from the normal anabolic storage state to one of catabolic breakdown. There is a greatly increased energy expenditure, leading to raised nutritional requirements, which are further increased by, for example, stress, anxiety, heat loss, dressing changes and anaesthetics. In a burn of 50% body surface area, the basal metabolic rate may double, this change persisting until the patient is virtually healed. To maintain the energy supply, the body draws on all the available stores, including muscle.

Any trauma leads to a release of catecholamines, which act to increase the levels of circulating glucose, leading in turn to raised levels of insulin, glucagon, growth, hormone and glucocorticoids. Glucagon acts to increase gluconeogenesis, which is largely from the substrates of muscle breakdown and proteolysis, as fat is a relatively poor source of substrates. The excess nitrogen released is then excreted in the urine and can be used as a measure of protein breakdown. Maintaining adequate nutrition and calorie intake can reduce the amount of protein lost and prevent the gross wasting seen in some burns patients. Early feeding regimens and the nutritional aspects of treatment are discussed in greater depth in Chapter 9.

References

Batchelor ADR, Kirk J and Sutherland A (1961) The treatment of shock in the burnt child. *Lancet* (Jan): 123–127.

Baxter CR (1974) Fluid volume and electrolyte changes in the early post-burn period. *Clinics in Plastic Surgery* **1**: 693.

Baxter CR (1981) Guidelines for fluid resuscitation. *Journal of Trauma* **21**: 667.

Baxter CR and Shires T (1968) Physiological response to crystalloid resuscitation of severe burns. *Annals of the New York Academy of Science* **150**: 874.

Carvajal HF (1980) A physiological approach to fluid therapy in severely burned children. *Surgery, Gynecology and Obstetrics* **150**: 379–384.

Cope O and Moore FD (1947) The redistribution of body water and the fluid therapy of the burned patient. *Annals of Surgery* **126**: 1010–1045.

Davies JWL (1982) Prompt cooling of burned areas. A review of the benefits and the effector mechanisms. *Burns Journal* **9**: 1–6.

Demling RH (1987) Fluid replacement in burned patients. *Surgical Clinics of North America* **67**: 15–22.

Evans IE, Purnell OJ, Robinett PW et al (1952) Fluid and electrolyte requirements in severe burns. *Annals of Surgery* **135**: 804–817.

Frame JD, Eve MD, Hackett MEJ et al (1985) The toxic shock syndrome in burned children. *Burns* **11**: 234–241.

Harkins HN, Lam CR and Romence H (1942) Plasma therapy in severe burns. *Surgery, Gynecology and Obstetrics* **75**: 410.

Kyle MJ and Wallace AB (1951) Fluid replacement in burnt children. *British Journal of Plastic Surgery* **3**: 194.

Lawrence JC (1986) The causes of burns in burncare. A teaching symposium. Hull: Smith and Nephew Ltd.

Lawrence JC (1987) British Burns Association recommended first aid for burns and scalds. *Burns Journal* **13**: 153.

Lawrence JC (1966) First aid measures for treatment of burns and scalds. *Journal of Wound Care* **5**: 319–322.

Lund CC and Browder NC (1944) *Surgery, Gynecology and Obstetrics* **79:** 352.

Monafo WW (1970) The treatment of burns shock by intravenous and oral administration of hypertonic lactate solution. *Journal of Trauma* **10:** 575.

Moncrief JA (1972) Burn formulae. *Journal of Trauma* **12:** 538.

Moyer CA (1953) An assessment of the therapy of burns. *Annals of Surgery* **137:** 628–638.

Moyer CA, Margraf HW and Monafo WW (1965) Burn shock and extravascular sodium deficiency – treatment with Ringer's solution with lactate. *Archives of Surgery* **90:** 799–811.

Muir IFK (1961) Red cell destruction in burns. *British Journal of Plastic Surgery* **14:** 273.

Muir IFK and Barclay TL (1962) Treatment of burn shock. In Muir IFK and Barclay TL, *Burns and their Treatment*, pp 14–54. London: Lloyd-Luke.

Reiss E, Stirman JA, Artz CP et al (1953) Fluid and electrolyte balance in burns. *Journal of the American Medical Association* **152:** 1309–1313.

Settle JAD (1974) Urine output following severe burns. *Burns* **1:** 23–42.

Settle JAD (1982) Fluid therapy in burns. *Journal of the Royal Society of Medicine* **75**(1): 1–11.

Underhill FP, Carrington GL, Kapsinov R and Pack GT (1923) Blood concentration changes in extensive superficial burns, and their significance for systemic treatment. *Archives of Internal Medicine* **32:** 31–48.

Wilson GR and French G (1987) Plasticised polyvinyl chloride as a temporary dressing for burns. *British Medical Journal* **294:** 556–557.

Wilson GR, Fowler CA and Housden PL (1987) A new burn assessment chart. *Burns* **13:** 401–405.

Further Reading

Cason JS (1981) *Treatment of Burns*. London: Chapman & Hall.

Clarke JA (1992) *A Colour Atlas of Burn Injuries*. London: Chapman & Hall.

Muir IFK, Barclay TL and Settle JAD (1987) *Burns and their Treatment*. London: Butterworth.

5

Wound Care

This chapter outlines the normal processes of wound healing and how the ability of the skin to repair itself depends on the depth of skin damage. The initial care and treatment of the burn wound are described, with particular attention to certain anatomical areas. Infection control procedures are briefly considered throughout. Finally, the care of less extensive/minor wounds is discussed.

The healing process and the immune response are natural occurrences and are completely automatic. They do not depend upon medical care; on the contrary, medicine depends on them.

When one imagines a patient suffering from severe burns, it is difficult to comprehend that the body has the ability to repair itself. In these cases, without medical intervention, the complications caused by hypovolaemia and septicaemia would be fatal long before the stages of the healing process were able to take place. According to Cason (1981), it would take months or even years for a 30% full thickness burn to heal spontaneously, and the patient would have succumbed to infection or complications long before.

However, patients suffering from less extensive injuries are able to heal naturally, which is well demonstrated by a partial thickness burn. Deeper burns will also be capable of the physical and biochemical processes of healing, but at a prolonged rate and with a poor cosmetic appearance.

Scientific knowledge has allowed surgeons to save lives by the excision of necrotic tissue and the application of skin grafts. This reduces the risks of infection, promotes healing and returns the skin's natural protective function. Surgical intervention also offers an improved cosmetic appearance over that of a deep burn left to heal by its own devices.

Research into the processes of wound healing has resulted in the development of wound care products that facilitate the body's natural healing action. Therefore, whether a wound is to be treated surgically or conservatively with dressings, the best method of healing can be achieved. The wound care market is constantly developing new products; these continue to be clinically evaluated in Burns Units today.

THE STAGES OF WOUND HEALING

These stages are based upon the phases described by Westaby (1985).

Stage 1: Inflammation (0–3 days)

The phase of traumatic inflammation begins within a few minutes of injury and lasts for about 3 days. The features of this phase are similar to those caused by a wound infection, and care must therefore be taken not to confuse the two.

There are five classic signs of inflammation:

- Heat
- Redness
- Swelling
- Pain
- Loss of function

The signs of infection are as those given above, but with the addition of mal-odour, purulent exudate, green slough and extending cellulitis (Morison, 1994).

When tissue is damaged, the redness and heat are caused by the increased blood supply and cellular activity in the affected area. Injured blood vessels bleed into the defect until clotting occurs. Damaged tissue and mast cells secrete histamine and other enzymes that cause vasodilation and increased capillary permeability. The capillary walls then allow inflammatory exudate (containing plasma, anti-bodies, white blood cells and a few red blood cells) to infiltrate the surrounding tissues, resulting in swelling and oedema.

During this phase, two important cell types arrive at the wound site: polymor-phonucleocytes and macrophages. These defend against bacteria, and clear debris, damaged tissue and blood clots, thus leading to Stage 2.

Stage 2: Destruction (2–5 days)

The wound is cleaned of devitalised tissue by the polymorphonucleocytes and macrophages. Macrophages are large mobile cells that can engulf and digest bacteria and dead tissue. They play a crucial role in the process of wound healing, for if they are removed healing ceases (Westaby, 1985). This is because they attract further macrophages to the wound site, where they are responsible for stimulating the development and multiplication of fibroblasts. Fibroblasts synthesise collagen, which is the supportive fibrous protein of the skin.

Macrophages are also known to initiate angiogenesis, the process by which new blood vessels are formed; these vessels grow into the wound from the edges, and fibroblasts follow them to assume their role. This is the beginning of Stage 3. The natural degradation of devitalised tissue is known as autolysis and requires a moist environment to promote its occurrence (Davis et al, 1993).

Stage 3: Proliferation (3–24 days)

Fibroblasts begin to produce strands of collagen, the main constituent of connective tissue. The optimum environment for this to occur is one of slight acidity (Westaby, 1985). The production of collagen increases the tensile strength of the wound; early collagen is, however, irregularly constructed, and its synthesis depends upon the vascularity and perfusion of the wound. Vitamin C and lactate ions are crucial stimulators for this stage, and collagen synthesis is inhibited if the nutritional intake of vitamin C is insufficient. Most of the factors that impair healing during this phase are systemic; they include age, anaemia, hypoproteinaemia and zinc deficiency (Westaby, 1985).

The activity of the healing process at this stage produces granulation tissue, consisting of new and fragile capillary loops supported in a scaffolding of collagen fibres. The granulation tissue is moist, red and fragile, and it fills the wound, allowing it when combined with the processes of epithelialisation and contraction to heal. The wound will, at the end of this stage, have the appearance of being healed but will remain red, raised and itchy.

Stage 4: Maturation (24 days–1 year)

During this phase, the structure of the new scar is extensively remodelled. There is a progressive decrease in the vascularity of the scar, and its red appearance fades. The amount of collagen initially increases but, after several months, reduces, flattens and softens. The strength of the scar gradually grows, although only 50% of the normal tensile strength of a skin wound is regained in the first 6 weeks (Westaby, 1985). Eventually, however, the scar will reach a strength comparable to that of normal tissue (Davis et al, 1993).

The time scales described at the beginning of each stage act only as a guide for a wound undergoing a simple healing process without complication. The time taken for many wounds to heal depends on a multitude of intrinsic and extrinsic factors, including their depth, size and chronicity, but they will still pass through these phases. Wounds can also have different stages of healing occurring at the same time. In addition to the four phases described above are the processes of epithelialisation and contraction, which are of greatest importance when there has been tissue loss or destruction, as in a burn injury.

Contraction

Contraction is the process by which large wounds become small without the need for a skin graft or secondary closure (Westaby, 1985).

The mechanism of contraction is not yet fully understood, but certain facts are known (Westaby, 1985).

- Collagen is not essential
- Myofibroblasts supply the motive force

- Interference with the viability of cells at the wound edge inhibits the process
- Contraction can begin on the fourth day after injury

Epithelialisation

The skin has a covering of squamous epithelial cells that are constantly being shed and replaced from below. When an injury causes a defect in this squamous covering, the cells at the wound edges multiply, flatten and migrate towards the area of cell deficit (Westaby, 1985). This mechanism is of vital importance after a burn injury, as it is the major factor in deciding whether or not the burn will require a skin graft (see below).

Wounds epithelialise not only from the wound edges but also from deep dermal appendages that are lined with epithelium, such as hair follicles (Figure 5.1). Epithelialisation can begin within hours of injury during the inflammatory phase, but the cells will only migrate over live tissue and will move into the layer below debris, blood clots or eschar (Figure 5.2).

In the wounds allowed to heal by this method the protective influence of a scab or dressing prevents physical trauma, drying, haemorrhage and invasion from micro-organisms. In order for the fragile epithelial cells to migrate across the wound surface, a moist environment under a non-adherent dressing is preferable, as it facilitates the process (Davis et al, 1993; Westaby, 1985). Owing to the intense cellular activity in the area, the wound edges have a raised hyperplastic zone, which disappears once epithelialisation is complete. The process ceases when the epithelial cells meet across the wound surface by 'contact inhibition' (Pape, 1993).

LOCAL PATHOPHYSIOLOGY OF THE BURN WOUND

Heat causes injury to the cells, resulting in tissue destruction and seriously impairing the normal functioning of the skin. The interruption of the protective barrier that the skin provides leaves an accessible route for micro-organisms to enter the body's internal environment. Life is then threatened by this vulnerability to infection and the overall systemic effects to the circulation.

The burn wound has been described as having three zones (Dyer and Roberts, 1990), which are three-dimensional, as demonstrated by Figure 5.3 (Rylah, 1992).

1. The zone of *coagulation* – usually in the centre of the wound, compromising of non-living tissue.

2. The zone of *stasis* – tissue is viable but, having decreased perfusion and, is at risk of ischaemic damage.

3. The zone of *hyperaemia* – normal skin with increased blood flow as a response to injury.

When a burn injury occurs, the body responds by initiating the inflammatory

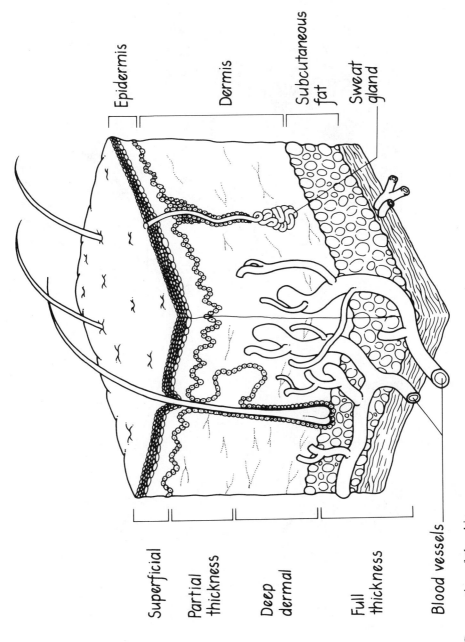

Fig 5.1 Cross-section of the skin

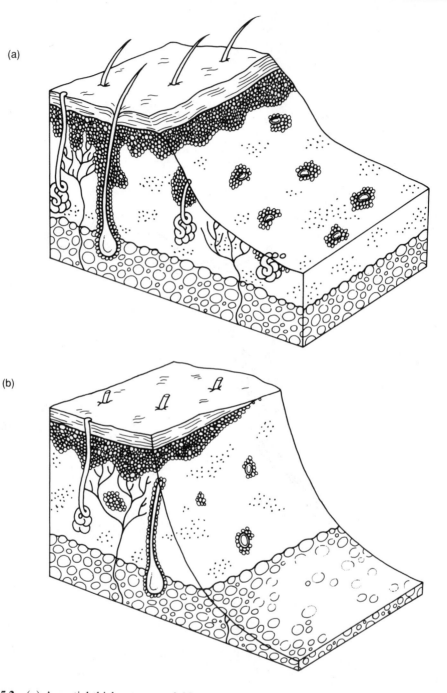

Fig 5.2 (a) A partial thickness wound. Numerous islands of epithelium remain around the hair shafts and glands each being a source of regeneration. (b) A full thickness round. No viable epithelium remains in the wound area; dermis heals slowly by granulation and a skin graft may be needed.

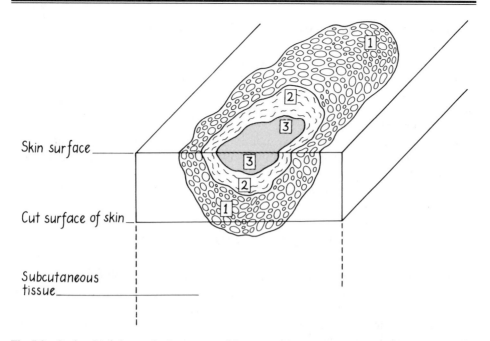

Skin surface

Cut surface of skin

Subcutaneous
tissue

Fig 5.3 Pathophysiology of a burn wound 1: zone of hyperaemia; 2: zone of stasis; 3: zone
of necrosis

process, as described above. Burn oedema formation is rapid and produces copious
amounts of exudate. In order to stop the burning process, immediate care of the
burn is to cool it with cold water. This reduces, and can even reverse, the total
cellular damage and oedema formation (Clarke, 1992).

The inflammatory process is completed as the oedema subsides, and the series
of events that follows is as in the healing process described above.

However, the ability of the skin to repair itself depends on the depth of skin
damage, which is an important factor in determining treatment.

BURN DEPTH AND THE HEALING PROCESS

The assessment of the depth of tissue damage does not take place until 48 hours
post-burn injury, when the oedema has subsided. Wound healing and management
will vary, depending on the type of burn, and many injuries will be a combination
of different depths. Superficial burns, involving only the epidermis, and partial
thickness burns, involving the upper layers of dermis, have the ability to heal spontaneously in approximately 7 to 14 days respectively (Clarke, 1992). This is possible because the damage only extends to the mid-dermis, and the deep dermal
appendages, such as hair follicles and sweat glands, remain intact. As described
above (Figure 5.2a), because these are encapsulated by a layer of epithelial cells

that can regenerate, the wound can heal by itself and the result is only minimal scarring.

Deep partial thickness/deep dermal burns involve the majority of the dermis, leaving only the deepest layers intact. Some of the dermal appendages will remain, but epithelialisation will be slow, healing will be prolonged over 3–4 weeks and poor-quality skin cover will result (Parker, 1993).

Full thickness burns involve all the layers of the skin and may extend to fat, muscle, tendon and bone. Granulation and contraction are the processes by which these wounds heal, with epithelialisation only occurring from the edges in the latter stages (Figure 5.2b). This can take weeks or months and will leave unsightly scarring.

Deep partial thickness and full thickness burns will therefore benefit from excision and skin grafting.

CARE OF THE BURN WOUND

At the scene of the injury, the first aid measures should be followed by application of a clean, non-fluffy material to protect the burned area from further contamination. 'Cling-film' is ideal (Wilson and French, 1987); otherwise, a clean sheet can be used. Elaborate dressings are inappropriate, and ointments should not be applied as they hamper subsequent wound assessment (Settle, 1986).

On arrival at the Accident and Emergency Department, although it is the appearance of the damaged skin that is most shocking, it is the treatment of the airway, breathing, circulation and pain that takes priority over any wound procedure.

Once these functions have been stabilised and the body surface area covered by the burn has been assessed, care of the wounds can then begin. It is essential that the dressing technique incorporates strict asepsis to try to prevent any contamination of an already immunocompromised patient. The wearing of an apron and sterile gloves for the nurse, and sterile towels to surround and cover the patient, assist in maintaining a clean environment.

Management of the Wound

The burn wound is irrigated with warmed normal saline (Clarke, 1992) to prevent further cooling of the wound site and the patient. Dead epithelium is trimmed away using sterile scissors and forceps, and blisters are deroofed. Most physicians choose to evacuate and debride the blisters covering large burns because the fluid they retain may increase the risk of infection by acting as a culture medium for bacteria; additionally, the roof of the blister will degrade to slough after a few days (Rockwell, 1990). Blisters also impede the assessment process and can restrict movement if they are over joints, so only small blisters are left intact. Any foreign material, such as clothing and debris, will need gently removing from the wound, and it may be necessary to wash away any soot or dirt with tap water and non-perfumed soap (Parker, 1993). Hair in the close vicinity of the wound may also require clipping, as it will become encrusted with exudate and act as a focus for bacterial colonisation. When the wound has been assessed, further treatment can if necessary, take place.

Circumferential Burns

An important consideration before the wound dressing is applied is whether or not the burn appears to be circumferential around the neck, chest, limbs or fingers, particularly if it already appears to be full thickness (Settle, 1986). As the burn oedema develops, the inelastic eschar acts as a tourniquet and has the potential to cause fatal ischaemia of the extremities, or respiratory difficulty if the chest or neck is constricted. If this complication arises, the tension created by the restricting eschar must be released by an escharotomy. This is a longitudinal excision through the burned skin along its full extent, and, because the skin is dead, no analgesia is required (Settle, 1986). An alginate dressing with haemostatic properties is applied to the escharotomy site, as the relief of tension causes the wound to gape open and some bleeding will occur when viable tissue is reached.

Dressing the Burn Wound

The objective of applying dressings to a burn injury is to prevent colonisation of the wound by pathogenic bacteria, to absorb exudate and to provide a moist environment for wound healing.

Paraffin gauze is the primary dressing of choice when initially covering a large area of burn (Settle, 1986). It is relatively inexpensive, and when several layers are placed upon a heavily exudating wound, it has a low adherence to the wound surface because it remains moist. Layers of gauze followed by gamgee pads are then applied to the wound to absorb the prolific amounts of exudate. Crêpe bandages are used to hold the dressings in place. As soon as any leakage occurs through the bandage layer, there is a route by which micro-organisms can enter the wound from the environment, and repadding is required (Parker, 1993).

When lengths of paraffin gauze and cotton gauze are applied to the limbs or the chest, they should not be wrapped around in spirals as they will act as a tourniquet when the oedema is maximal. Crêpe bandages are used because they will stretch to accommodate for swelling, but the patient should be regularly checked for any discomfort. The neck is an area that is unable to have a bandage applied, so a paraffin gauze collar is made and held in place by a rolled-up gamgee in a tubular gauze stocking or a physiotherapy collar, to keep the chin elevated.

Burned limbs and extremities should be elevated to minimise the swelling that will occur from the formation of oedema, and, for the same reason, patients with burned faces should be nursed in an upright position.

In the Nottingham Burns Unit, the type of dressing described above is applied for the first 48 hours of treatment, until the assessment of wound depth is made. No creams are initially applied, because of their tendency to 'mask' the wound, causing it to appear deeper than it actually is. The assessment of burn depth is of great importance at this time, as it influences the decision of whether surgical intervention will be necessary.

There are five anatomical areas that are an exception to this treatment: the face, ears, hands, feet and perineum.

Face

Burned faces are regularly cleaned with warmed saline and are then left exposed until they are dry and the exudate has coagulated. Soft paraffin may be applied over any crusted areas to facilitate easy removal of dead skin and to moisturise the new epithelium. Partial thickness burns treated by exposure should start to shed their coagulum after 12 days, revealing healed skin underneath. Attempts to remove any scabs before they are loose will damage the developing epithelium underneath. When the surface of a full thickness burn separates, a dressing or skin graft may be required (Settle, 1986). Soft white paraffin is applied to the lips to prevent cracking and soreness, which may inhibit nutritional intake, and oral hygiene must be attended to with regular mouth and dental care. A patient who has suffered facial burns will usually have shut his eyes during the accident as an automatic reaction, except in extreme circumstances. Eyelashes will be singed, diminishing the protection that they normally provide, and the eyes will be susceptible to infection. The eyes are initially checked for damage with fluorescein eye drops (Cason, 1981); they are then kept clean and moist with regular applications of normal saline. It is imperative that the patient is warned that his eyes will close as a result of the oedema, and emphasis should be placed upon the fact that this is only temporary.

Ears

When ears are burned, it is important that the cartilage is not allowed to dry out, as this can lead to deformity. If any infection occurs to the ears, this can cause internal damage and result in complications and defects of hearing. For these reasons, silver sulphadiazine cream is applied (after the ears have been gently plugged with paraffin gauze), and paraffin gauze and cotton gauze padding is held on by a head bandage or netting bonnet.

Hands and Feet

If the digits of hands and feet are burned, it is preferable for their movement to be maintained, to prevent the stiffening and contraction of joints. Silver sulphadiazine cream is applied, and the hand or foot is placed in a Goretex bag. Goretex has replaced the use of plastic bags as a dressing, as it allows gaseous exchange to take place through it and prevents the wound becoming macerated (Muddiman, 1989; Martin, French and Theakstone, 1990). If the arm, leg or digit has a circumferential burn, a plastic bag will still be used, so that the hand or foot can be observed for signs of decreased circulation, such as pallor, coolness, numbness and lack of pulses.

Perineal Burns

In both males and females, the oedema resulting from a burn to the perineum may obstruct or impede the passing of urine. Catheterisation may consequently be required in the initial stages of treatment before swelling occurs. The perineum is again a site with an increased risk of infection owing to the close proximity of the anus and the urethra. The area is dressed with paraffin gauze and padding, which is changed each time the patient uses the toilet, meticulous attention being paid to hygiene.

These dressings are all continued until the 48-hour 'check'. When the wounds have been properly assessed, silver sulphadiazine cream may then be applied to all the areas, in conjunction with the paraffin gauze.

1% silver sulphadiazine cream has a broad-spectrum antibacterial effect and is particularly effective against Gram-negative organisms such as *Pseudomonas aeruginosa* (Settle, 1986). The cream needs to be applied every 24–48 hours in order to achieve its therapeutic effect, and it helps to achieve a moist environment conducive to wound healing (Parker, 1993). As the risk of septicaemia is so great in patients suffering from major burns, wound swabs are obtained for microbiological culture and sensitivity at each dressing change. However, when the wounds have mostly healed, and in the case of minor burns, it is only necessary to take a wound swab if signs of infection are present or infection is suspected. Wound infection should always be treated with a systemic antibiotic rather than topical preparations (Morison, 1994).

Wound Care of Minor Burns

After the initial period of maximal exudation is over (at around 48 hours) the wound, if it is small enough to be managed in the Outpatient Department, may be dressed accordingly and the patient discharged home.

If a patient has a full thickness burn but is unfit for or refuses surgery, the necrotic tissue or eschar will have to be removed by wound care products that have been designed for that purpose, for example by the use of an enzymatic debrider or a hydrogel to rehydrate the eschar. Hydrocolloid dressings can also be used to rehydrate small areas of necrotic tissue. Wounds, when kept warm and moist, will debride themselves by the process of autolysis described above.

Granulating wounds and epithelialising wounds require a warm, moist environment to heal under a non-adherent dressing. Hydrocolloids are widely used in the Nottingham Burns Unit for this purpose, although they are unsuitable for heavily exuding wounds. They provide an ideal healing environment for a partial thickness burn after the exudate has subsided, as they can be left undisturbed.

One problem with the burn wound is that it has a tendency to overgranulate, which is when the granulation tissue rises above the surrounding skin level before the wound has achieved epithelial cover. This is treated with a steroid cream, under paraffin gauze and a padded dressing.

In conclusion, the aim of the overall treatment and care of the burn wound is to control the proliferation of bacteria on the burn surface, to provide a moist environment to promote healing, to encourage the separation of burn eschar and eventually, to achieve a clean, vascularised wound bed that will heal spontaneously or will accept a skin graft.

References

Cason JS (1981) *Treatment of Burns*. London: Chapman & Hall.
Clarke JA (1992) *A Colour Atlas of Burn Injuries*. London: Chapman & Hall.
Davis H, Dunkley D, Harden R et al (1993) *The Wound Handbook*. Dundee: Centre for Medical Education.
Dyer C and Roberts D (1990) Thermal trauma. *Nursing Clinics of North America* **25**(1): 85–117.
Martin DL, French GWG and Theakstone J (1990) The use of semi-permeable membranes for wound management. *British Journal of Plastic Surgery* **43**: 55–60.
Morison MJ (1994) *Which Wound Care Product*. Professional Nurse Information Sheet. London: Austin Cornish.
Muddiman R (1989) A new concept in hand burn dressing. *Nursing Standard*, Supplement, September 23, 1–4.
Pape SA (1993) The management of scars. *Journal of Wound Care* **2**(6): 354–360.
Parker JA (1993) *Burns Educational Leaflet No. 14*, Part 1. Northampton: The Wound Care Society.
Rockwell W (1990) Should burn blisters be burst? *Emergency Medicine* **22**(11): 57–59.
Rylah LTA (1992) *Critical Care of the Burned Patient*. Cambridge: Cambridge University Press.
Settle JAD (1986) *Burns. The First Five Days*. Romford: Smith & Nephew.
Westaby S (1985) *Wound Care*. London: Heinemann.
Wilson GR and French G (1987) Plasticised polyvinyl chloride as a temporary dressing for burns. *British Medical Journal* **294**: 556–557.

6

Care of the Burns Patient

with an Inhalation Injury

Despite advances in the fluid resuscitation, wound management and metabolic support of the burn-injured patient, inhalation injury still remains a strong determinant of survival.

The severity of smoke inhalation was first appreciated in the 1942 Cocoanut Grove nightclub fire in Boston (Mass.), in which 491 people died, many of whom appeared to have minimal injuries. An autopsy study of the fire victims revealed that 70% of patients who died within 12 hours of admission had a documented inhalation injury (Zikria et al, 1972).

Although there are no national statistics available in the UK, it is thought that the mortality attributed to inhalation injury ranges from 45 to 90% of admissions, depending on the reporting institution.

Inhalation injury is the leading cause of death in the first 24-hour period after a burn (Harvey et al, 1984). Early diagnosis and aggressive pulmonary support are vital to patient survival, providing an important challenge to the burns multidisciplinary team.

PRE-HOSPITAL CARE

As in all aspects of trauma, the initial treatment is vital, and the priorities at the scene of the accident must remain the same. The airway must be assessed, breathing established and the circulation confirmed to be adequate for vital cell functioning. Oxygen must be given if there is any suspicion or evidence of inhalation injury. The ideal is 100% oxygen, preferably delivered via a tight-fitting mask. Establishing information at the scene of the accident can aid later diagnosis (Table 6.1).

ACCIDENT AND EMERGENCY DEPARTMENT CARE

Immediate assessment must be made to determine or alleviate an inhalation component of the injury. A very quick visual assessment must continue (Table 6.2).

Table 6.1   Initial assessment of inhalation injury: the history

- Was there an explosion, i.e. gas or chemicals?
- Was the fire in a confined space, e.g. car or building?
- Was the patient trapped inside a confined space for a period of time?
- Was the patient conscious on removal from the scene of the accident?
- What products, e.g. wood, plastic or wool, were burning?

Table 6.2   Clinical features of inhalation injury

- Is the face burnt?
- Is the neck burnt? Is it circumferential (i.e. may require escharotomy)?
- Are the nasal hairs singed?
- Is the patient coughing up carbonaceous sputum?
- Is the oral or pharyngeal mucosa inflamed?
- Is there any hoarseness of the voice?
- Is there any difficulty in breathing or stridor?
- Is the patient disorientated or confused?

Airway obstruction due to oedema may develop very quickly, so if doubt exists, the airway should immediately be secured with a good size (7 mm or above in adults) endotracheal tube; failure to do this could be catastrophic. Communication between the Accident and Emergency Department and the specialist unit is very important, in order to discuss treatment and to organise the safe transfer of the patient as soon as priorities have been dealt with (See Chapter 4).

MECHANISMS OF INJURY

Upper Respiratory Tract

External burns to the face and neck can lead to massive oedema in the first 24-hour period, making airway management difficult, if not impossible, if early treatment is not correctly undertaken.

The need for escharotomy of the neck and chest should be assessed, and the procedure should be performed once the airway is established.

The upper airway attempts to protect itself from hot, dry air by reflex opening and closing of the glottis, to protect against brief exposure to heat. Each breath has the capacity to cool air down from a possible 500°C to 50°C before it reaches the carina (Moritz et al, 1945).

Heat exposure is usually caused by the inhalation of hot gases, which, when in contact with the cells lining the respiratory tract, cause tissue injury, producing a very quick inflammatory reaction. Oedema can occur rapidly, resulting in severe narrowing of the airway. A similar reaction can occur on ingestion of corrosive liquids, such as bleach or caustic soda, and even in accidents with children scalding their mouth or pharynx with hot water (Mathur, 1986).

Table 6.3 Respiratory irritants and asphyxiants and their effects

Toxicant	Source	Water solubility	Effects
Ammonia (NH$_3$)	Wool, silk, nylon	High	Unbearable odour
Chlorine			Mucosal irritant
Hydrogen	Polyvinyl chloride (plastics), furniture, retardent treated materials	High	Respiratory irritant
Acetaldehyde Formaldehyde Arolein	Wallpaper, acrylic lacquered wood, cotton	Low	Mucosal damage, extensive lung damage
Cyanide	Any combustible products		Headaches
Carbon monoxide	Polyurethane, nylon upholstery, paper		Tissue hypoxia Narcosis

Lower Respiratory Tract

The added presence of smoke to hot gases increases the degree of injury quite dramatically. Smoke consists of irritant particles, mainly of carbon, which can vary in size and are deposited in the respiratory tree. Toxic chemicals are produced by the incomplete combustion occurring in fires, depending on what is burning. These chemicals can be arranged into two broad categories; irritants and chemical asphyxiants. Some irritants are identified in Table 6.3, the major asphyxiants being carbon monoxide and cyanide.

These irritant gases and particulate matter can have a severe cytotoxic effect. It is the water solubility of the compound that determines the degree and location of cellular injury. Highly water-soluble toxic gases dissolve rapidly on the first moist surface they encounter, which tends to be the upper airway. Gases with low water solubility tend to injure the lower respiratory tract and lung parenchyma (Cioffi and Rue, 1991).

Airway damage continues from the upper airway ulceration and inflammation, to further cell death and sloughing. The oedema can be compounded by a massive fluid resuscitation requirement. Smoke and toxicants may have damaged alveolar epithelium and capillary endothelium, and there could also be a ciliary paralysis, which could lead to bronchospasm, small airway plugging, a deficiency of surfactant and subsequent atelectasis. Increased humidity can also cause severe thermal pulmonary damage extending to the distal bronchioles (Heimbach and Waeckerle, 1988).

Steam, which is essentially air at 100% humidity and at least 100°C, has a heat-carrying capacity approximately 4000 times that of air (Peters, 1981). Although steam burns can directly injure the lung, they are fortunately rare.

Toxic Fumes

Carbon Monoxide

Carbon monoxide (CO) is a tasteless, colourless, non-irritatant gas, a byproduct of the incomplete combustion of organic materials (Meridith, 1988). It is released into the air during fire and explosions and can cause the percentage of oxygen to decrease from 21 to less than 10 in that situation (Crappo, 1969).

It is because of carbon monoxide's affinity for haemoglobin, which is 200–250 times that of oxygen, that it remains the greatest killer at the scene of an accident. The binding of carbon monoxide to haemoglobin also shifts the oxygen disociation curve to the left (Douglas et al, 1912), thereby further decreasing the blood's ability to deliver oxygen to the tissue.

The historical 'cherry pink' presenting colour of the carbon monoxide poisoned patient is rare. The effects of acute carbon monoxide poisoning depend on its concentration in the environment, the activity level of the victim and the duration of exposure (Burney et al, 1982). For example, lethal concentrations of carbon monoxide from car exhaust fumes can be reached in a closed car garage in 10 minutes (Stewart, 1975).

Oxygen in high concentration is given to the patient as early as possible (including at the scene of accident and in transit to hospital), in order to compete for haemoglobin binding sites (although caution should be taken in patients with chronic lung disease).

It must be remembered that blood samples taken at the time of admission to hospital will not provide an accurate exposure picture. Clarke et al's (1981) normogram permits the calculation of carboxyhaemoglobin levels from the time of exposure, starting from a measured concentration, to a known time interval up to 5 hours post-exposure. It shows that carboxyhaemoglobin levels of 30–45% can be expected with severe inhalation injury, and that these patients will still have levels of 20–25% 3 hours after exposure. Mathur (1986) states that it would be normal to presume that a carboxyhaemoglobin level of 15% 3 hours post-injury is strong evidence of smoke inhalation.

The normal carboxyhaemoglobin level varies depending on whether the person is a smoker or non-smoker, but a level of greater than 1.5% in a non-smoker and greater than 5% in a smoker should alert one to the likelihood of upper airway damage (Robinson and Miller, 1986). A co-oximeter capable of directly measuring carboxyhaemoglobin is a valuable asset to a Burns Unit.

A comparison of carboxyhaemoglobin levels and the clinical symptoms associated with these can be seen in Table 6.4.

Hyperbaric Oxygen

This is quoted as the treatment of choice for severe carbon monoxide poisoning, although facilities in the UK are few and far between. Therapy comprises of the intermittent inhalation of 100% oxygen at a pressure greater than that at sea level. This effectively displaces the carbon monoxide from haemoglobin, myoglobin and the cytochrome systems, improving the neurological status by maintaining viability

Table 6.4 Comparison of carboxyhaemoglobin levels and the associated clinical symptoms

Carboxyhaemoglobin (%)	Possible signs and symptoms
1–10	Normal range
10–30	Headache (throbbing), flushing, irritability
	Mild exertional dyspnoea, impaired vision
30–40	Dizziness, vomiting
40–50	Tachycardia, tachypnoea, fainting/collapse
>60	Coma, convulsions, cardiopulmonary arrest
80	Rapidly fatal

Table 6.5 Investigations used in confirmation of inhalation injury

- Bloods
  - carboxyhaemoglobin
  - arterial blood gases
- Chest X-ray
- Fibre-optic bronchoscopy
- ^{133}Xenon ventilation–perfusion lung scan
- Pulmonary function tests

of neurones in the ischaemic brain until circulation is restored by reducing the cerebral oedema (Bayley, 1991).

There is a fear that pulmonary damage is worsened, owing to the high levels of oxygen used, but Cianci and Sato (1994) consider it to be a comprehensive treatment significantly improving morbidity and mortality, and cost-effective in reducing patient stay.

Cyanide

Polyurethane foam, a modern furniture filler, gives off, when burning, a very dense black smoke, containing not only corrosive agents but also cyanide compounds, which may be lethal, as cyanide is a cellular poison. Cyanide fumes are rapidly absorbed through the skin and respiratory tract, and death occurs at a serum level of approximately 100 mmol/l.

Treatment of intoxication should focus on detoxification, early ventilation and hyperoxygenation, with aggressive treatment of metabolic acidosis.

SPECIALIST CARE IN THE BURNS UNIT

The treatment commenced in the Accident and Emergency Department is continued once the patient reaches the Burns Unit, and a full and thorough assessment is repeated by the plastic surgeons and anaesthetic and nursing staff. The prescribed treatment depends on the severity of the inhalation injury, but the overall aim is to maintain effective respiratory exchange until healing has taken place in the airways, and to reduce the risks of further complications, such as infection. After the initial clinical examination, investigation must continue to determine baselines and confirm any suspicion of inhalation injury. Some of these investigations (Table 6.5) may have been carried out in the Accident and Emergency Department but, depending on results, may be repeated.

Investigations

Blood Samples

- Carboxyhaemoglobin levels (see Table 6.4 above)
- Arterial blood gases: these may be normal on admission and should be repeated if there is a clinical indication.

A low partial pressure of arterial oxygen (PaO_2) (less than 10 kPa when the inspired oxygen concentration is 50%; i.e. $FiO_2 = 0.5$) is suggestive of an inhalation injury.

Arterial blood gas level is an important tool for the continued assessment of patients with brain or suspected inhalation injury (Moylan, 1981).

Chest X-Ray

A standard chest X-ray taken within the first 24 hours has not been found to be an early sensitive indicator of inhalation injury (Puttman et al, 1977), but at approximately 48 hours, there appears to be a relationship between the degree of X-ray change and pulmonary function (Peitzman et al, 1987), which coincides with clinically important pulmonary dysfunction (increased extravascular lung water volumes, increased intrapulmonary shunt function or decreased compliance).

Fibre-optic Bronchoscopy

This is the most helpful diagnostic tool, allowing immediate diagnosis of laryngeal or tracheobronchial mucosal inflammation, oedema, necrosis, ulceration and soot in the airways (Cioffi and Rue, 1991).

Cioffi and Rue (1991) recommend that bronchoscopy is performed once fluid resuscitation commences, so that impaired bronchial blood flow secondary to hypovolaemia does not provide vasoconstriction, obscuring mucosal changes and producing a false negative result. This technique, in which a flexible fibre-optic bronchoscope is passed into the trachea via either the nasal or oropharyngeal route, can be performed at the bedside, with minimal risk to the patient. If endotracheal intubation has already been carried out, the bronchoscope can be passed down this tube. If not, it can be passed down the nose, pharynx and larynx following anaesthetisation with lignocaine.

133Xenon Ventilation–Perfusion Lung Scan

This is helpful in diagnosing injury to the small airways and lung parenchyma, but must be carried out within the first 24–48 hours post-injury. After this period of time, a false negative result may occur, as the hyperventilation associated with thermal injury may accelerate the washout of xenon from the injured lung tissue (Cioffi and Rue, 1991).

[133]Xenon isotope is injected intravenously into the patient, and serial scintiphotograms are obtained to identify the pulmonary clearance of the isotope. A normal study shows no trapping of the isotope and a complete washout within 90 seconds. Inequality of the elimination pattern, however, is suggestive of pulmonary parenchymal injury (Lund et al, 1985).

Pulmonary Function Tests

It is believed that normal spirometry results exclude the diagnosis of significant inhalation injury (Sataloff and Sataloff, 1984), but there appears to be no difference in lung volume between patients with and those without inhalation injury. Patients with inhalation do, however, show an increase in the work of breathing (Stephenson et al, 1975) because of increased pulmonary resistance (Nyhus, 1983).

A combination of bronchoscopy, xenon scintigraphy and pulmonary function testing yields a 90% accuracy in the diagnosis of inhalation injury and essentially eliminates false negative results (Agee et al, 1976). The present author, however, thinks it unlikely that many Burns Units in the UK would have access to all these facilities or the desire to complete all the tests for diagnosis.

To summarise, diagnosis of inhalation injury investigations are there to support and confirm initial suspicions, which start with clinical examination and the history.

Airway Management

Oxygen Therapy

All patients in whom there is suspicion or evidence of inhalation injury will require oxygen therapy, the aim being to deliver oxygen to the hypoxic tissues.

The oxygen must be humidified, as normal mucosa may be damaged. The nose, usually our natural humidifier, warming and filtering inspired air, is often ineffective at this stage. The humidification will also help pulmonary secretions to retain moisture, facilitating the effective clearing of tenacious secretions.

Patients should sit upright (which will also help to reduce facial oedema), be given chest physiotherapy, and be encouraged to deep breath and cough to expectorate if possible, any secretions. Bronchodilators are used for the treatment of bronchospasm and wheezing.

The indications for the use of oxygen therapy are given in Table 6.6.

Table 6.6   Indications for oxygen therapy

- Carbon monoxide poisoning
- PaO_2 < 10 kPa and low arterial oxygen saturation (SaO_2)
- Changes in mental status – cerebral hypoxia
- Peripheral cyanosis due to hypotension and hypovolaemia
- Central cyanosis due to obstruction or inhalation damage

Mechanical Ventilation

The indications for mechanical ventilation for an inhalation injury are the same as those for any trauma patient: upper airway obstruction, copious amounts of thick secretions that are inadequately cleared, and acute pulmonary insufficiency. Criteria more specific to burns that are commonly used are (Bartlett et al, 1976):

- Smoke inhalation followed by coma
- Respiratory depression
- Nasolabial full thickness burns
- Circumferential neck burns
- Burns of the upper airway confirmed by fibre-optic bronchoscopy

Airway

1.   *Endotracheal*   The artificial airway route of choice is a nasotracheally placed endotracheal tube, and, to facilitate adequate removal of the secretions, this must be at least 7 mm in diameter in an adult. Nasal alar necrosis can occur, so nursing care must be meticulous, ensuring regular checks on the tension and direction of the tube and the attached piping. If a large-volume, low-pressure variety of tube is used, it can stay in place for up to 3 weeks, after which tracheostomy must be considered.

2.   *Tracheostomy*   This is avoided where possible, owing to the associated morbidity – tracheal stenosis, ulceration, tracheoesophageal fistula and direct contamination of the airway from the burn surface (Moylan, 1980). Table 6.7 is a comparison between endotracheal and tracheostomy tubes.

   If oxygen therapy alone is unable to maintain effective respiratory function, intermittent positive pressure ventilation (IPPV) is required. Ineffective gaseous exchange is identified by the arterial blood gas picture and a mixture of symptoms (Table 6.8). High fractions of inspired oxygen may initially be necessary to achieve oxyhaemoglobin saturations of over 90%, and relatively high tidal volumes may be needed to reduce the risk of atelectasis.

Positive End-expiratory Pressure (PEEP)

If the PaO_2 remains low even with these high fractions of oxygen, PEEP is indicated, as it improves the ventilation of the poorly or non-ventilated segments of the lung, thus preventing alveolar collapse. The goal is that oxygenation can be

Table 6.7 Comparison of endotracheal and tracheostomy tubes

Type of tube	Advantages	Disadvantages
Endotracheal	• Non-surgical insertion	• Risk of nasal–alar cartilage damage
	• Easy removal	• Hard to secure in the presence of facial burns and oedema
	• Decreased bacterial contamination of the lungs	• Communication difficult – patient is unable to mouth words
		• Must be changed after 3 weeks owing to risk of laryngeal damage
Tracheostomy	• Easier pulmonary toilet	• Direct access for infection (especially if neck burnt)
	• Easy fixation of tube	• Risk of tracheal stenosis
	• Greater patient comfort/tolerance	• Risk of tracheoesophageal fistula
	• Greater potential for communication	

Table 6.8 Ineffective gaseous exchange

Ineffective gaseous exchange can be detected by:
- $PaO_2 < 8$ kPa, with FiO_2 of 0.5
- $PCO_2 > 7.5$ kPa and rising
- Decreased pH
- Increased pulse rate
- Decreased respiratory rate
- Cyanosis
- Irritability

maintained at an FiO_2 of 0.5 or less, as high concentrations of oxygen can be toxic to the lungs. The usual pressure range employed is 0.5–1.5 kPa (5–15 cm H_2O).

The benefits of PEEP can, however, be counterbalanced by decreased cardiac output and an increased risk of barotrauma, for example pneumothorax and pulmonary interstitial emphysema. It may also lead to increased fluid retention in the lung in the patient with pulmonary oedema.

Continuous Positive Airway Pressure (CPAP)

A constant gradient of distending pressure is applied to the spontaneously breathing patient via an endotracheal tube, tracheostomy or tight-fitting mask. It can be used in acute respiratory failure or in the weaning process prior to extubation.

Intermittent Mandatory Ventilation (IMV)

IMV allows for spontaneous breathing between 'mandatory' ventilator-delivered breaths. The mandatory component is reduced as the patient's ability to increase his spontaneous minute volume improves. Sedation can be reduced and a muscle relaxant avoided, allowing the weaning process to be initiated.

Synchronised IMV (SIMV) allows the patient to 'trigger' a breath, but if no breath is 'triggered' within a predetermined time period, a mandatory breath is automatically determined.

Weaning from a Ventilator

If ventilation has been continued for several weeks, weaning can be both difficult and slow, and it should be attempted only when the patient has recovered sufficiently to regain adequate ventilatory and pulmonary reserves. The chest X-ray and PaO_2 on an FiO_2 of less than 30% should be normal. SIMV can be helpful followed by CPAP, as the patient's respiratory function allows.

Vital signs, arterial blood gas levels and respiratory variables must be closely monitored, observing for signs of distress or exhaustion.

Secretion Clearance

Frequent and meticulous tracheobronchial toilet must be carried out, using strict aseptic technique. A catheter should be introduced gently into the trachea and withdrawn, applying intermittent rotating suction over a period of about 15 seconds. If oxygen desaturation occurs, a self-sealing endotracheal tube adaptor should be used.

Chest physiotherapy, postural drainage of respiratory secretions and manual hyperinflation 'bagging' of the lungs with 100% oxygen pre- and post-suctioning are crucial to the care of the patient.

Drug Therapy

Antibiotics

Prophylactic systemic antibiotics are not advocated, except in paediatric burn patients, as their use may serve only to hasten the selection of antibiotic-resistant organisms (Levine et al, 1978).

Wound swabs, sputum specimens and urine and blood cultures should be obtained if infection develops, so that the offending organism can be identified and the appropriate antibiotics used (Pruit et al, 1975).

Steroids

Steroids appear to be contraindicated in patients with an inhalation injury and body surface area burn, owing to their immunosuppressant effects. Complications and morbidity are significantly increased.

Steroids have been shown to:

- Reduce lung bacterial clearance, resulting in increased risk of infection (Sataloff and Sataloff, 1984)
- Promote wound healing (Trunkey, 1978)
- Promote mechanical breakdown of the trachea in intubated patients (Moylan and Alexander, 1978)

Additionally, they have been shown to be of little or no value in smoke inhalation injury alone (Demling and Lalonde, 1989).

Bronchodilators

Bronchodilators have been advocated to relax bronchospasm and aid the reduction of swelling (Chu, 1981). Salbutamol may be given via a nebuliser and aminophylline by intravenous infusion or as a bolus injection.

Stress Ulcer Prophylaxis

In a study of ventilated patients receiving stress ulcer prophylaxis, it was found that sucralfate had decreased mortality rate, and reduced positive findings of bacteria and bacterial concentrations in the stomach (Tryba, 1987).

The oropharynx, stomach and digestive tract have been recognised as important endogenous sources of micro-organisms that may potentially lead to pneumonia. Thus, selective decontamination of the digestive tract of the critically ill, ventilated patient is an attempt to decrease bacterial colonisation, and therefore translocation of these bacteria, by the administration of oral, parenteral and topical antibiotics to the oral cavity is suggested (VanSaene and Stoutenbeck, 1987).

Monitoring

Respiratory Function

Chest X-Ray

Although abnormalities may not be seen immediately post-injury, serial studies thereafter may be requested to indicate a progression of the effects of inhalation injury and the response to treatment.

Pulse Oximetry

This is an effective means of monitoring peripheral oxygen saturation and perfusion on a continuous, non-invasive basis. Pulse oximetry responds rapidly to hypoxia and degrees of desaturation that could be undetected clinically, especially during suction or repositioning of the patient.

Arterial Blood Gases

Initially arterial blood gas readings may be unremarkable, especially in upper air-way damage, but they can provide an important baseline. Abnormal arterial blood gases may indicate injury to the lower airway. In the ventilated patient, any adjust-ment or change to the ventilator parameters should be followed after approximately half an hour by an arterial blood gas analysis, as it is the most accurate means of assessing adequate oxygenation, carbon dioxide elimination and acid–base status.

Hypoxia may result from any combination of alveolar damage, ventilatory insuf-ficiency, circulatory impairment and oxygen transport derangement, for example increased carboxyhaemoglobin levels.

PCO_2 is usually normal in the early stages but may rise later, and metabolic acidosis owing to tissue hypoxia is often found.

Carboxyhaemoglobin Levels

The presence of high carboxyhaemoglobin levels is an indication of carbon monoxide poisoning and its need for, or response to, treatment (see the section on carbon monoxide poisoning above).

Fibre-optic Bronchoscopy

Assessment can be made on the progression of oedema, mucosal sloughing and overall upper airway damage, and used as an aid to reassessment and treatment.

Cardiovascular Function

Monitoring should include pulse, arterial blood pressure and continuous electro-cardiogram readings, but the use of invasive monitoring, requiring the insertion of either a central line or a Swan–Ganz catheter, should be avoided if possible, as the complications of insertion are much greater in the burns patient.

Central Venous Pressure (CVP)

In the severely compromised patient presenting with particular haemodynamic problems, for example heart failure or septicaemic shock, CVP measurement is useful. It is a direct measure of the state of hydration of the patient, and, in hypo-volaemic shock, can give an indication of the adequacy of fluid replacement and an early warning of overloading.

The normal value CVP lies between 3 and 5 cm H_2O, but it must be remem-bered that positive pressure ventilation will increase the CVP by 8–12 cm H_2O.

Swan–Ganz Catheterisation

The Swan–Ganz catheter is a balloon-type catheter inserted via a CVP approach into the right pulmonary artery via the right atria; it is necessary for the close monitoring of pressures, blood gases and cardiac output.

The pulmonary artery wedge pressure (normally 5–15 mmHg) is a measurement that when done on a serial basis, guides the management of fluid therapy, and could also indicate the need for inotropic support. It is a useful measurement in patients with adult respiratory distress syndrome, left ventricular failure and low serum albumin.

Cardiac output can be measured by a volume of cold saline being injected into the pulmonary artery and its dilution, as measured by a thermistor in the catheter tip, being estimated. A mini-computer presents the data as cardiac output, and the infusion rates of the inotropes can be adjusted accordingly.

Metabolic and Fluid Balance

Regular weight and attention to strict fluid balance are important. Blood should be taken for full screening, including hepatic and renal investigations, and other values, for example haemoglobin, packed cell volume, white cells, platelets and clotting factors, should be closely monitored.

Complications

Respiratory Infection

Infection from damaged skin or other organisms may cause tracheobronchitis or bronchopneumonia and the treatment for the infection is determined by culture of the sputum. Treatment can, however, sometimes commence prior to this on the clinical picture of the patient alone.

Adult Respiratory Distress Syndrome (ARDS)

Although known to many of us as ARDS, other names, for example stiff lung, shock lung, wet lung, ventilator lung and post-traumatic pulmonary insufficiency, are now also commonly used.

The characteristics are that of respiratory distress: dyspnoea, tachypnoea, cyanosis, diffuse pulmonary infiltration of chest X-ray, reduced pulmonary compliance and a marked increase in alveolar/arterial oxygen difference. Fine crepitations can also be heard in both lung fields.

There is likely to be a low PaO_2 despite oxygen administration, tachycardia and an increased respiratory rate. Pulmonary oedema will persist, a hyaline membrane forms, and there is ultimately interstitial pulmonary fibrosis, obliterating the pulmonary architecture, including the microvasculature. This all results in reduced lung compliance, and gross hypoxaemia can develop insidiously 24–72 hours post-trauma.

Possible causes of ARDS in the burns patient are:

- *Infection* – septicaemia associated with skin breakdown, pneumonia
- *Inhalation* – from smoke, corrosive agents, resulting in loss of surfactant, or oxygen toxicity, resulting in the formation of a hyaline membrane, which leads to a failure of gaseous exchange

- *Aspiration* – of gastric acid
- *Haematological* – after massive blood transfusion, especially of unfiltered blood, with microaggregates causing multiple microemboli in the lungs, or as a result of disseminated intravascular coagulation
- *Metabolic* – renal failure

Mortality from ARDS is high and is attributed to multiorgan failure from sepsis, rather than to hypovolaemia per se (Montgomery et al, 1985; Petty, 1985).

CASE STUDY

Harry is a 59-year-old man admitted with 20% body surface area burns to face, neck, hands and, in patches, on his legs. He was also diagnosed in the Accident and Emergency Department as having an inhalation injury.

The Scene of the Accident

It is thought that Harry poured petrol over a settee and set fire to it in the early hours of the morning. The Fire Service was called when his wife realised that the lounge was on fire. Harry was removed from the burning lounge and given 15 litres of oxygen via a mask. He was conscious.

The Accident and Emergency Department

Owing to the facial burns, the history of the accident and a carboxyhaemoglobin level of 34% on admission, it was decided to intubate Harry with a size 9.0 mm endotracheal tube.

He was given etomidate and atracurium for the intubation, and thereafter fully ventilated. Transfer was arranged to the Intensive Care Unit (not all Burns Units have the facilities to ventilate patients).

Intensive Care Unit

Day One   On initial examination Harry's chest was clear, but there was evidence of black soot seen at the back of his throat and in secretions in the endotracheal tube. He was given a bronchoscopy, results confirming that large amounts of soot covered all his airways and that his mucosa was inflamed. Lavage was attempted but had little effect. Harry's ventilation was on the SIMV mode, with a tidal volume of 800 ml, a respiratory rate of 13 breaths per minute, a PEEP of 7 and the oxygen decreased from 100 to 60%. No respiratory effort was made at this stage.

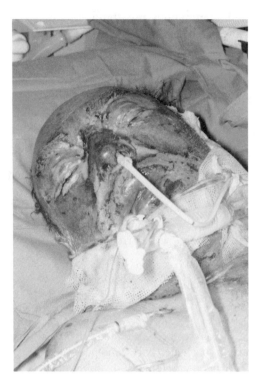

Fig 6.1   Harry in the Intensive Care Unit approximately 12 hours after admission

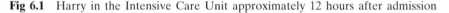

Day Two   Harry became cardiovascularly unstable, with a systolic blood pressure of 60 mmHg. A Swan–Ganz catheter was inserted so that cardiac output studies could be performed, and inotropic support (dobutamine and noradrenaline) was given. Secretions at this stage were thick and soot-stained, and Harry's chest sounded 'crackly'.

Arterial blood gas levels and oxygen saturations were borderline, but Harry was rapidly developing pulmonary oedema. Copious amounts of watery, frothy secretions were coming from his chest, and the FiO$_2$ had to be increased to 90%. Intravenous frusemide was given via a continuous infusion.

Day Three   Harry's chest had very audible bilateral crepitations and copious secretions.

Day Six   Harry's condition was much more stable, so consideration was given to weaning him off the inotropes and removing the Swan–Ganz catheter. Weaning off ventilation also commenced by adding an assisted spontaneous breathing component of 20 (or pressure support) to the SIMS rate at 40% oxygen.

Day Nine   The assisted spontaneous breathing component was now reduced to 10, with an FiO_2 of 40% and a CPAP of 4.

Day Ten   Bronchoscopy was repeated; there was still gross inflammation of the main airway, an oedematous larynx and evidence of thick, sooty secretions. The inotropes were discontinued.

Day Eighteen   The FiO_2 was decreased to 30%, and Harry was weaned off assisted spontaneous breathing. He was making a good respiratory effort, and a T-piece was considered next.

Day Nineteen   The T-piece was in situ, and Harry was self-ventilating and maintaining an oxygen saturation of 94% on 40% oxygen.

Day Twenty-five   A tracheostomy was performed, and Harry was transferred back to the Burns Unit.

The Burns Unit

The insult to Harry's airway was severe. Heat from the fire had damaged the upper airway, and carbon particles had damaged the lower airways. Although careful fluid balance had been implemented, pulmonary oedema had still developed. Diuretics were used to remove the excess fluid, and inotropic agents were used to maintain tissue perfusion.

Harry required a tracheostomy, owing to the fact that the secretions were still present in such large quantities and Harry was unable to clear them independently, so they were forming a barrier to effective gaseous exchange.

Weaning Harry off the ventilator took a long time, but this is often the case. Multiple operating theatre attendances for skin grafting are just one of the circumstances that lead to the ventilation mode being changed.

A few minutes longer in the smoke-filled room, or inappropriate medical/nursing management, could quite easily have been fatal for Harry. As it was, Harry made a good recovery (Fig. 6.2). However, sadly, Harry died in July 1996. This was not related to the incidents described above.

SUMMARY

In order to improve the management of an inhalation injury in the burn injured patient Bartlett (1979) suggests the goals of treatment in seven steps.

1.   Try to avoid lung oedema
2.   Maintain normal pulmonary capillary integrity by avoiding factors known to cause pulmonary capillary leakage and ischaemia

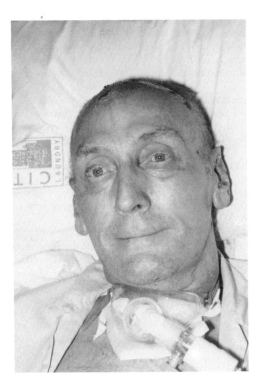

Fig 6.2   Harry on the road to recovery, with tracheostomy tube in situ

3. Avoid infection
4. Minimise fibrosis by minimising oedema
5. Avoid hypoventilation
6. Provide adequate monitoring
7. Maintain airway clearance

References

Agee RN, Long JM III, Hunt JL et al (1976) Use of 133 Xenon in early diagnosis of inhalation injury. *Journal of Trauma* **16**: 218.

Bartlett RH (1979) Types of respiratory injury. *Journal of Trauma* **19**: 918–919.

Bartlett RH, Niccole M and Travis MJ (1976) Acute management of the upper airway in facial burns. *Archives of Surgery* **111**: 744.

Bayley EW (1991) Care of the burn patient with an inhalation injury. In: Trofino RB (ed.) *Nursing Care of the Burn Injured Patient*, pp 325–348. Philadelphia: FA Davis.

Burney RE, Wu SC and Nemiroff MJ (1982) Mass carbon monoxide poisoning: clinical effects and results of treatment in 184 victims. *Annals of Emergency Medicines* **18**: 394–399.

Chu C (1981) New concepts of pulmonary burn injury. *Journal of Trauma* **21**: 958–961.

Cianci P and Sato R (1994) Adjunctive hyperbaric O_2 therapy in the treatment of thermal burns: a review. *Burns* **20**(1): 5–14.

Cioffi WG and Rue LW (1991) Diagnosis and treatment of inhalation injuries. *Critical Care Clinics of North America* **3**(2): 191–198.

Clarke CJ, Campbell D and Reid WH (1981) Blood carboxyhaemoglobin and cyanide levels in fire survivors. *Lancet* **1**: 1332–1335.

Crappo RO (1969) Smoke inhalation injuries. *Journal of the American Medical Association* **246**: 1694.

Demling RH and Lalonde C (1989) *Burn Trauma*, pp 3–23. New York: Thieme.

Douglas CG, Haldane JS and Haldane JBS (1912) The laws of combination of haemoglobin with CO and O_2. *Journal of Physiology* **44**: 275–304.

Harvey JS, Watkins GS and Sherman RT (1984) Emergency burn care. *Saith Medical Journal* **77**: 204–214.

Heimbach DM and Waeckerle JF (1988) Inhalation injuries. *Annals of Emergency Medicine* **17**: 1316–1320.

Levine BA, Petroff PA, Slade CL et al (1978) Perspective trials of dexamethasone and aerosolized gentamicin in the treatment of inhalation injury in the burned patient. *Journal of Trauma* **18**: 188.

Lund T, Goodwin CW, McManus WF et al (1985) Upper airway sequelae in burn patients requiring endotracheal intubation or tracheotomy. *Annals of Surgery* **201**: 374.

Mathur NK (1986) Inhalation injury in major burns. *Care of the Critically Ill* **2**(5): 195–196.

Meridith T (1988) Carbon monoxide poisoning. *British Medical Journal* **296**(6615): 77–78.

Montgomery AB, Stager MA, Carrico J and Hudson LD (1985) Causes of mortality in patients with adult respiratory distress syndrome. *American Review of Respiratory Disease* **132**: 485–489.

Moritz AR, Henriques FC and Mclean R (1945) The effects of inhaled heat on the air passages and lung: an experimental investigation. *American Journal of Pathology* **21**: 311–331.

Moylan JA (1980) Smoke inhalation and burn injury. *Surgical Clinics of North America* **60**: 1533–1540.

Moylan JA (1981) Inhalation injury: a primary determinant of survival following major burns. *Journal of Burn Care and Rehabilitation* **3**: 78–84.

Moylan JA and Alexander GJ (1978) Diagnosis and treatment of inhalation injury. *World Journal of Surgery* **2**: 185–191.

Nyhus LM (1983) Current treatment of the extensively burned patient. *Annals of Surgery* **15**: 331–364.

Peitzman AB, Shires GT, Texider HS et al (1989) Smoke inhalation injury: evaluation of radiographic manifestations and pulmonary dysfunction. *Journal of Trauma* **29**: 1232–1239.

Peters JW (1981) Inhalation injury caused by the products of combustion. *Canadian Medical Association Journal* **125**: 249–252.

Petty TL (1985) Indicators of risk, cause and prognosis in adult respiratory disease. *American Review of Respiratory Disease* **132**: 485–489.

Pruit BA Jr, Ereckson DR and Morisa A (1975) Progressive pulmonary insufficiency and other pulmonary complications of thermal injury. *Journal of Trauma* **15**: 369–379.

Puttman CE, Loke J, Matthay RA et al (1977) Radiographic manifestations of acute smoke inhalation. *American Journal of Roentgenology, Radium Therapy and Nuclear Medicine* **129**: 865–870.

Robinson L and Miller RH (1986) Smoke inhalation injuries. *American Journal of Otolaryngology* **7**: 375–380.

Sataloff DM and Sataloff RT (1984) Tracheostomy and inhalation injury. *Head and Neck Surgery* **6**: 1024–1031.

Stephenson SF, Esrig BC, Polk HC and Fultan RL (1975) The pathophysiology of smoke inhalation injury. *Annals of Surgery* **182**: 652–660.

Stewart RD (1975) The effect of carbon monoxide in humans. *Annual Review of Pharmacology* **15**: 409–422.

Trunkey DO (1978) Inhalation injury. *Surgical Clinics of North America* **58**: 1133–1140.

Tryba MD (1987) Risk of acute stress, bleeding and nosocomical pneumonia in ventilated intensive care patients: sucralfate versus antacids. *American Journal of Medicine* **83:** 117–123.

VanSaene HKF and Stoutenbeck CP (1987) Selective decontamination. *Journal of Antimicrobial Chemotherapy* **20:** 462.

Zikria BA, Weston GC, Chodoff M et al (1972) Smoke and carbon monoxide poisoning in fire victims. *Journal of Trauma* **12:** 64.

7

Management of Pain

in the Burns Patient

The degree of pain experienced by people who have sustained burn injuries varies greatly. It depends not only on the severity of the actual tissue damage and the individual's response to pain but also on the type of treatment he or she is receiving. It is because of these many factors that the level of discomfort will constantly change, unless appropriate methods of pain control are used and evaluated.

The need for analgesia during the initial treatment is often minimal, even though the injuries may be severe. This is because when the patient has sustained full thickness burns, the sensory end organs have been damaged and have lost the ability to detect and transmit pain impulses. Conversely, this does not mean that individuals who have partial thickness burns are constantly in agony. It is sometimes necessary to touch burned areas of the patient in order to assess the severity of the injury. This is measured by the response when light pressure is applied with a sterile needle to the affected areas (pinprick test). A positive response will indicate that the sensory end organs are at least partially functioning. However, the patient may not be in a great deal of pain when no procedures are being carried out. It is worth noting that those who suffer superficial burns will have their sensory end organs intact and may therefore suffer a great deal of pain.

Any area of the skin that has lost the protective outer layer will have exposed nerve endings that will be sensitive to both the atmosphere and the application of any form of dressing. The level of discomfort at this stage can be reduced by applying a layer of plasticised polyvinyl chloride ('Cling-film') over the wounds to exclude the air. This form of covering will enable the wound to be assessed without the need to remove conventional dressings, which are painful to remove and time-consuming to apply, and may damage some healthy tissue when frequently applied and removed during the assessment stage. 'Cling-film' is an ideal covering during both the assessment and transit stages and can remain in situ until an appropriate dressing is applied (Wilson and French, 1987).

When an individual has a burn injury, he rarely sustains the same degree of burn all over his body so most patients will suffer varying levels of pain. This becomes apparent when they try to move or when pressure is applied to particular areas. Many patients do not suffer a great deal of pain until health professionals become involved, which is when patients least expect to experience pain. Most patients expect pain or discomfort to be diminished in a care setting, therefore the carer must consider anticipating pain levels, so that the appropriate action can be taken.

WHAT IS PAIN?

In order to take appropriate action, the nurse must understand what pain is and what the word pain means to the individual.

Pain is a complex, distressing experience, involving sensory, emotional and cognitive components. The word 'pain' is derived from the Greek word 'poire' meaning punishment. The International Association for the Study of Pain (1986) gives the following definition:

Pain is an unpleasant sensory and emotional experience with actual or potential tissue damage. Each individual learns the application of the word through experiences related to injury in early years.

Pain is experienced by almost every patient who has sustained a burn injury. Although patients who have sustained severe burns present with many problems, pain is often their most significant complaint. Therefore, the assessment, prescription and administration of effective analgesia are of paramount importance.

Burns nurses are in an ideal position to assess and evaluate the management of pain; their unique role, and the amount of time they spend in direct contact with the patient, means that they are ideally placed to advise the medical staff on the effectiveness of analgesia regimens.

Studies of orthopaedic patients have shown that prolonged pain can increase the period spent in hospital and prevent patients from attaining their full potential, because they are unwilling or unable to fully participate in the rehabilitation phase of their recovery (Crocker, 1986). By promoting communication between all members of the multidisciplinary team, in order to co-ordinate painful procedures and give effective analgesia in advance, the intensity and frequency of pain can be reduced to a minimum. To do this effectively, the patient's day must be planned and the level of discomfort assessed over a 24-hour period. In so doing, discomfort is reduced and patient co-operation increased, thus obtaining the optimum level of recovery for the individual.

The nurses' perception of pain can become dulled because of their frequent exposure to suffering. There is also a tendency to associate a particular level of discomfort or pain with different procedures or degrees of trauma, which is evidently not so. There appears to be little or no correlation between the severity of the injuries sustained and the pain experienced.

This also demonstrates that pain and discomfort are very much individual experiences. It is necessary therefore to adopt an operational definition of pain and have a clear understanding of our aims when managing people in pain.

It is helpful to take McCaffery's (1979) statement of what pain is to the individual and adapt this to create a working aim:

Pain is whatever the experiencing person says it is, existing whenever he says it does.

The **aim of care** is *to learn to observe and listen to the patient, to recognise the level of physical and emotional pain being felt, and then to help to reduce this pain to a minimum.*

This aim takes into consideration the many factors that affect the level of discomfort that an individual experiences. However, it also emphasises that the nurse should be forming a partnership with the patient, using his or her knowledge, understanding and expertise to reduce the pain as much as possible.

FACTORS THAT INFLUENCE PAIN

There can be no doubt of the benefits of reducing any pain to a minimum. However, although each individual will feel and display discomfort in different ways, there are many common factors that can affect the severity of pain, which must be considered in patient management.

The factors that influence the severity of pain are:

- The depth of the burn
- The percentage of body surface area burnt
- Other injuries
- Analgesia already administered
- The manner of the initial management
- The psychological response to injury
- Fear and anxiety
- Previous painful experiences

So that the pain can be reduced to a minimum, and because even people with the same injuries may react differently to the stress of trauma, nurses must individualise their methods of pain management. Patients' diverse reactions therefore require the team to be aware of, and be prepared to use, a variety of methods of pain control. For this reason, the amounts of psychological support and analgesia required will never be the same.

Factors such as age, gender and the cultural background of the patient will affect the way he reacts to pain. It is sometimes difficult for people to express their feelings and fears with someone of another gender or from a different cultural background, which will be magnified if there is a communication problem owing to the inability of nurses to understand the patient's language. These problems can be overcome by the use of an interpreter and by ensuring that staff receive appropriate cultural awareness training. Establishing simple common signs, or the use of a picture board with symbols that demonstrate discomfort, the severity of the pain and the need for analgesia, can go some way to solving this. Once the picture board has been made, the patient simply points to the relevant symbol to make his wishes known. A system similar to this can be used with patients who have endotracheal tubes in situ.

THE RATIONALE FOR ADDRESSING THE PROBLEM
OF PAIN MANAGEMENT

If adequate pain relief is not initially achieved, the patient begins to anticipate pain every time a member of the burns team attempts to carry out a procedure, whether or not it is potentially painful. This can result in poor patient co-operation and an increasing tendency towards dependence, because the patient is afraid to move for fear of experiencing pain. This is one of the main contributing factors for burns patients becoming increasingly demanding. The problem of pain management must be addressed as soon as the patient arrives on the unit. Pain itself can act as a barrier between the patient and members of staff, because a patient in pain is unlikely to communicate freely with carers. Staff members can actively work towards reducing this barrier by effectively reducing the level of discomfort and keeping the patient fully informed about what is happening. Hayward (1979) demonstrated that information given to the patient actively decreases anxiety levels, and therefore reduces the amount of pain felt.

In order for us to be able to assess and manage pain effectively, we must have an understanding of the factors that affect the perception of pain in the individual. We must also be aware of the different types of pain and how this 'pain' is transmitted and interpreted by the body (the mechanism of pain).

The pain experienced by an individual post-burn injury will change during progression through the phases of recovery. Initially, there may be acute pain that has had a rapid onset giving individuals no time to prepare themselves; there will also be a time during this phase when they will have had no analgesia. The individual may also have been denied emotional or psychological support if the injuries were sustained in an isolated area.

After this initial phase has passed, the patient is at the beginning of the long road to recovery via planned treatment and rehabilitation. He will have to undergo many painful procedures, often resulting in unpredictable levels of discomfort. This stage may last for some time, as it is not unusual for burn patients to be receiving some kind of therapy months and even years after their accident. The type of pain felt during the different stages of treatment will vary and can present the team with different management problems. Some of this pain can be anticipated, for example during the following activities:

- Clinical examination
- Clinical procedures, for example the insertion of intravenous lines
- Dressings/wound care
- Surgery
- Physiotherapy
- Mobilisation
- Daily living activities, for example eating, dressing and washing

It is this planned discomfort that can be reduced to a minimum by increasing the knowledge and understanding of pain and pain management. By looking at the factors that influence pain, and establishing which ones are variable, staff can

Table 7.1   Factors affecting the pain threshold

Threshold lowered	Threshold raised
Discomfort	Relief of symptoms
Insomnia	Sleep and rest
Fatigue	Sympathy
Fear and anxiety	Understanding and companionship
Mistrust	Trust
Anger, sadness and depression	Diversional activities
Boredom and introversion	Reduction in anxiety
Mental isolation	Elevation in mood
Social abandonment	Analgesics and antidepressants

work with the patient to reduce the level of pain as much as possible. Hayward (1979) clearly demonstrated that information reduces anxiety levels and thus reduces the level of post-operative pain; therefore, we must be honest with patients and actively work to keep them as informed as possible about future treatments and their possible side-effects, such as pain or discomfort. Alternative methods of pain control can be discussed, and the patient can take an active part in his own care. In entering into a partnership with the patient, one can strive to ensure that the resuscitation and rehabilitation stages of treatment are pain-free.

THE WAY THE BODY REACTS TO PAIN

To achieve pain-free therapy, one must have a greater understanding of the way in which the body reacts to pain. Everybody has a different pain threshold, but each individual's pain threshold is affected by the same factors, which may lower or raise the threshold, and which must be considered when planning pain management. Some of these factors are included in Table 7.1.

THE ANATOMY AND PHYSIOLOGY OF PAIN

It is very difficult to manage pain effectively without a good knowledge and understanding of the mechanisms and theories of pain.

The Pain Mechanism

The structures that enable us to feel pain are the receptors (nociceptors), which are sensitive to painful stimuli. The impulse pathways (routes) carry the impulses to the interpreting centres, the areas of the brain that decode and act on these impulses. There is also an analgesic system that modulates and controls pain.

Pain Receptors

The concentration of pain receptors (nociceptors) varies greatly within the body, but they are found in nearly all tissue types. The nerve fibres are small and non-myelinated. Stimulation of the nerve endings results in the release of kinins. The rate of release is increased in the presence of prostaglandins, which themselves are released by damaged cells as part of the inflammatory process.

Pain Stimuli

A variety of agents either physical or chemical, can become stimuli, and the degree of stimulation felt is directly proportional to the intensity of the agent applied. Thus for heat, the higher the temperature, the greater the stimulus.

Pain Impulse Pathways

These are the paths or routes along which the impulses travel to reach the spinal cord or brain stem. They are made up of small (non-myelinated) and large (myeli-nated) nerve fibres, myelin being a fatty insulating sheath. When impulses travel along both types of fibres, we are aware of pain, but the sensation produced is different. Impulses travelling along the non-myelinated fibres travel slowly, producing the throbbing, dull, burning type of pain, whereas when impulses travel along the myelinated fibres, they travel at speed, creating the sharp, stabbing, localised pain often linked to an initial burns injury.

There are many theories that have been written to try to explain the physiology of pain, the two most common being the Specificity Theory and the Gate Theory. Using both theories together can explain most methods of pain control.

Theories of Pain

The Specificity Theory

This theory proposes that specific structures, namely nerve fibres, central nervous system pathways and neurones, are responsible for the passage of information to the brain. The areas that are covered by similar systems are pain, temperature, light touch and pressure. Impulses travel from the site of injury or stimulus via specific sensory nerve fibres to the spinal cord (first-order neurones), the route of entry to the spinal cord being via the posterior root ganglia and into the horn of grey matter. Many interconnections occur here, but most impulses travel to the brain via the spinothalamic tract (second-order neurones). These impulses travel through the brain stem to the thalamus (Figure 7.1a and b). The fibres related to pain and temperature terminate in the ventral posterior lateral nucleus of the thalamus where conscious recognition of pain and temperature occurs. From this point, the impulses are carried to the somesthetic area of the cerebral cortex by third-order neurones. This is where the pain is localised and, through past experience, the source of the pain identified. Pain is experienced when impulses reach the thalamus and brain stem, but interpretation of that pain is carried out in the cortex.

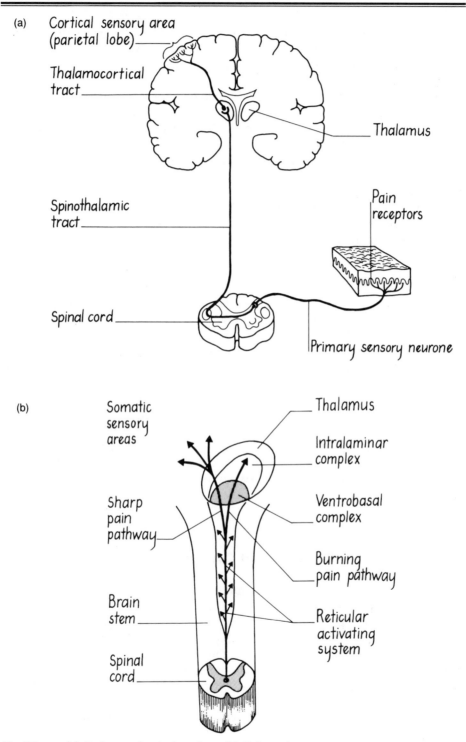

Fig 7.1   (a) Pathway of pain impulses. (b) Pain pathway.

The theory of specificity can be used to explain the benefits of the physical aspects of pain management, such as surgery, which can be used to sever or interrupt the pathway, thus stopping the passage of impulses.

Adjacent to the spinothalamic tract lies the anterior (ventral) spinothalamic pathway, which transmits nerve impulses relating to light touch or pressure. The touch fibres (mechanoreceptors) are located in the same areas of the skin as the pain receptors. It is these large, myelinated fibres that, when stimulated, close the pain gate and prevent pain impulses travelling up the spinothalamic tract. This is achieved by bombarding the first synapse with impulses, which explains why rubbing a painful area or applying transcutaneous nerve stimulation (TENS) is an effective method of managing pain.

However, not all impulses take this route; some are passed to the motor neurones at this first junction in the spinal cord. This process facilitates the instinctive or reflex-type reaction, for example removing the hand from a hot object.

The Gate Theory

The Gate Theory, initially proposed by Melzack and Wall (1965), suggests that there is an analgesic system within the brain and spinal cord that actively works to diminish the passage of pain impulses and thus reduce the level of discomfort experienced. The impulses carried to the spinal cord by the nerve fibres are blocked at their synapses in the posterior horns in the spinal cord. It is thought that this blocking is brought about by the action of a group of specialised neurones (the substantia gelatinosa) located close to each posterior column of grey matter.

The action of rubbing or the application of heat, or specifically in the case of burn injuries the cooling of the affected area, will produce increased activity in the large fibres. This increased activity 'closes the gate' on small fibres that carry the acute pain impulses. Conversely, increased activity in the small fibres 'opens the gate' and allows the impulses to pass to the posterior horn cells and on to the higher centres of the brain.

The Chemical Control of Pain

The pain control system is also susceptible to the effect of a variety of chemicals, some of which are produced naturally by the body and some of which are introduced into the body specifically to control the sensation of pain. These substances primarily work by suppressing or enhancing the passage of nerve impulses.

Endogenous chemicals (Table 7.2) form the basis of the body's analgesic system. When the body is under stress, it produces its own opiates, which can be generated by exercise, fear, excitement or a combination of all three. It is this process that enables people to continue physical exercise unaware of injuries they may have sustained. Because this system affects emotional status and mood, it can be used to rationalise the varied responses that different methods of pain control give rise to in different individuals.

Table 7.2 Endogenous chemicals affecting the sensation of pain

Name	Location	Function
Encephalins	Thalamus, hypothalamus, spinal cord pathways	Limit production of substance P
Endorphins	Pituitary gland	Limit production of substance P
Substance P	Sensory nerves, spinal cord pathways, areas of the brain involved with pain	Stimulates perception of pain
Serotonin	Brain stem	Alters sensory perception and mood

The previously mentioned theories of pain can be used to rationalise the use of the following methods of pain management:

- Distraction
- Local application of hot or cold substances
- Reduction in anxiety or fear
- Electrical stimulation (TENS)
- Acupuncture
- Analgesics (chemicals)

The passage of most pain impulses can be inhibited chemically at the synapses by analgesics. However, in some cases, it may be necessary physically to interrupt the pathway. Most forms of pain will respond to a combination of chemical and other therapies. Because of the variety of methods of controlling pain, it is essential to establish the most effective form of therapy for an individual patient at that particular time.

THE ASSESSMENT OF PAIN

In order to be able to decide what the best method of treating a particular type of pain is, it is necessary to understand as much as possible about the pain itself. This is a difficult task, because pain is a subjective experience. It is impossible to measure it in purely physiological terms, because of the psychological factors that influence the severity of pain or its importance to the individual. Therefore, the nurse must look beyond such factors as blood pressure, pulse and respiration rates.

In the acute stages of burn trauma management, it is helpful to look for ways of assessing and managing both the current and future physical and psychological pain. In this way, it is possible to plan pain relief to correspond with projected levels of pain.

When assessing a patient for the most effective methods of pain control, consideration must be given to the needs and goals of the patient and members of the burns team; in order to do this effectively, the patient needs to be assessed over a 24-hour period. This assessment takes into account the level of pain felt during physical therapy and also the pain endured at night. Both periods of the 24-hour day should be considered because they may present with very different management problems.

Pain is always difficult to measure, because it is only the person experiencing the pain who knows its nature, intensity and location. However, there are many guides that can be employed as an aid. These may take the form of a checklist, or they can include the use of tools to measure pain (McCaffery and Beebe, 1989). The use of assessment tools will promote a systematic approach to pain management and help to remove the subjective aspect. Appropriate tools are provided for the patients themselves to assess their pain, and this information should then be used in building up a complete picture, rather than being taken as a definitive value of pain. There is no one tool that is totally satisfactory for all patients, so an element of flexibility is required at all times.

One of the most frequently used tools is the Visual Analogue Scale (VAS) or linear scale (Huskisson, 1983). Such a scale is normally in the form of a 10 cm line, with the words 'No Pain' at one end, and 'Unbearable Pain' at the other. The user then describes the severity of the pain by pointing to the corresponding part of the line or stating the equivalent numerical value. A variation of this commonly used with children is the 'Pain thermometer', in which the range extends vertically from 0 (No Pain) to 4 (Unbearable Pain). Another system commonly used with children is a series of six pictures depicting a child in various degrees of discomfort (Figure 7.2).

Any such tools can prove helpful when looking at the intensity of pain, but it is necessary to be consistent once one has been chosen in order to prevent any misunderstanding.

VASs form a small but essential part of the construction of pain assessment charts. It is commonly acknowledged that the use of such charts should become

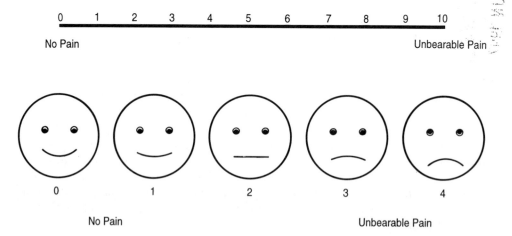

Fig 7.2   Examples of Visual Analogue Scales (VASs)

as routine as those for temperature, pulse and blood pressure. This is particularly important when dealing with victims of burn trauma or post-operative burn patients.

Pain assessment charts such as The London Hospital Pain Chart (Sharpe, 1986) can be adapted, especially for patients in Burns Units, to gain a better all-round picture of the pain.

To illustrate this, consider a young man who has sustained 22% burns to both hands, feet, face and left lower leg (Figure 7.3). He is 6 days post-burn, and has not, to date, required any surgery. He has, however, been experiencing a considerable amount of pain, particularly during dressing changes and physiotherapy. He has been on his present medication regimen for 48 hours. The mainstay of his analgesia is 30 mg of controlled release morphine tablets (MST Continus) twice daily. It is found that he requires additional analgesia for breakthrough pain; for this, dextromoramide (Palfium) is used, in conjunction with 50% nitrous oxide/50% oxygen (entonox) when necessary.

Using the chart, it is possible to plot a 24-hour profile of this patient's pain (Figure 7.4); the resulting pain profile or graph can then be used to adjust the type, dose and timing of any analgesia that is being administered. The profile can also be used to co-ordinate painful procedures; so that events such as dressing changes and physiotherapy coincide with the maximum effort to control the pain. The use of such charts can also be used to promote patients' involvement in managing their own pain. This is achieved by establishing what the optimum level of pain control is for the individual. When the profile is plotted, the patient can draw the optimal and maximum level of pain as horizontal lines on the graph. This then forms part of the plan to control pain. By observing the peaks and troughs of pain over a period of days, the analgesia regimen can be adjusted to achieve the optimum level of pain relief.

However, the importance of a thorough physical examination, an accurate history and a good understanding of the effects of pain on the patient cannot be overemphasised.

The following is a checklist of points to note when assessing a patient for pain:

1. Physical examination, to establish the source or cause of the pain.

2. Characteristics of the pain:

   - Type: crampy, sharp, stabbing, dull, throbbing, burning, etc
   - Intensity: mild or severe, on a scale of 0–10
   - Frequency
   - Duration
   - Changes in the site: tenderness, swelling and colour

3. Associated symptoms:

   - Nausea and vomiting
   - Altered level of alertness
   - Confusion or disorientation

4. The patient's priorities and aims.

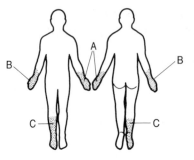

Date 15/4/94

Name Anon Anon

Age 21 years

Diagnosis 22% Burns

Linear scale for the assessment of pain

0 1 2 3 4 5 6 7 8 9 10

No pain   Unbearable pain

Time	Pain score				Analgesia		Activity/comments
					Type	Dose	
	A	B	C	Total			
0000	2	3	2	7			Watching television.
0200	0	0	0	0			Asleep.
0400	0	0	0	0			Asleep.
0600	4	6	5	15	MST	30 mg	Hands stiff/aching.
0800	6	6	3	15			Washing/eating. Dressing change.
1000	8	8	6	22	Palfium Entonox	20 mg 15 mins	Physiotherapy
1200	3	4	2	9			Eating.
1400	1	2	0	3			Visitors present, mind occupied.
1600	7	7	0	14	Palfium Entonox	20 mg 15 mins	Visitors leave. Physiotherapy
1800	4	3	1	8	MST	30 mg	Eating.
2000	2	1	1	4			Watching TV.
2200	3	2	2	7			Hands elevated in slings.

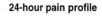

24-hour pain profile

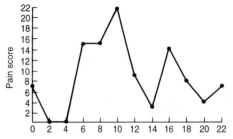

Plot total pain score/time to produce a 24-hour profile. This can then be used to assess the effectiveness of the action taken and assist in the planning of future management.

N.B. Compare 'peaks' of pain to activities carried out at any given time.

Fig 7.3 Pain assessment chart for burns

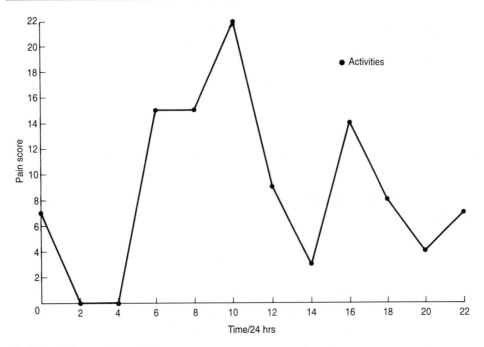

Fig 7.4   24 hour pain profile

ACHIEVING SUCCESSFUL PAIN CONTROL

The assessment of a patient in pain may take only seconds, perhaps on arrival in the Accident and Emergency Department. However, this is likely to be the beginning of a continuous period of assessment and the trial of a variety of methods until the goal of optimum pain relief is achieved.

The most widely recognised approach to pain management involves the use of a 'step-up' or 'ladder system'. This involves starting with mild non-opioids, and progressing to weak opioids and finally to strong opioids where necessary. It is not always practical when dealing with patients who are in pain as a result of burn trauma because the onset is often rapid and the pain frequently severe. However, once the pain is controlled, it should be possible to step down the analgesia ladder. This method will enable the pain to be controlled effectively using the most appropriate form and amount of analgesia.

If the patient is in pain immediately post-burn, the most effective form of analgesia is that achieved by opioids. These should administered intravenously and well diluted via a continuous infusion pump. Opioids should never be administered subcutaneously or intramuscularly immediately after a burn injury, because they will remain unabsorbed owing to the poor circulation. The danger is then that when the circulation improves and the opioids can be absorbed, the patient receives a large enough dose to depress the respiratory system. The regimen should be individualised and titrated against the patient's pain. It is generally recognised that there is no sealing dose if the patient remains in pain and is under close observation. Once a satisfactory level of pain control has been achieved, it is possible to reduce the dose to a maintenance level. It is often found that if good pain control is established early on in the treatment, the patient subsequently requires less analgesia.

ANALGESIC DRUGS IN COMMON USE

The most commonly used drugs involved in the management of pain fall into the categories given below.

Non-opioids

In this group are drugs such as paracetamol, as well as the non-steroidal anti-inflammatory drugs, for example ibuprofen and aspirin.

These drugs are usually found to be most effective on mild to moderate pain that originates in the musculoskeletal system.

Opioids

The term 'opioids' refers to any drug acting on the body's opioid receptors, for example morphine, diamorphine, codeine and dextromoramide.

Opioid drugs are used to relieve moderate to severe pain. Morphine and diamorphine have proved to be the most effective method of controlling pain in the initial stages of treating the burns patient. However, they need to be administered as a continuous infusion, preferably via a syringe driver.

Side-effects, such as a reduced respiratory rate, should not inhibit the use of this category of drug. However, patients receiving an opioid infusion should be monitored as frequently as their condition dictates. It is also necessary to assess the patient frequently with regards to the danger of constipation. The risk of dependence should not be taken into consideration when trying to control severe pain.

Local Anaesthetics

Local anaesthetics may be administered by injection or by the application of a cream or other agent directly onto the skin. EMLA cream is frequently used to site intravenous lines or for venepuncture on children. It must be applied at least one hour before the procedure is undertaken. EMLA has also been used when harvesting small split-skin grafts from adults, to obviate the need for a general

Table 7.3 Analgesics used for different degrees of pain

Drug	Form
Mild pain	
Ibuprofen	Tablet, liquid
Paracetamol	Tablet (soluble), liquid, Suppository
Aspirin	Tablet (Dispersible), Suppository
Moderate pain	
Coproxamol	Tablet
Codydramol	Tablet
Dihydrocodeine	Tablet, liquid, injection
Codeine phosphate	Tablet, liquid
Diclofenac	Tablet, suppository, injection
Entonox	Gas (50% nitrous oxide/50% oxygen)
Severe pain	
Pethidine	Tablet, liquid, injection
Morphine	Tablet, liquid, suppository, injection
Diamorphine	Liquid, injection
MST Continus	Tablet
Dextromoramide (breakthrough pain)	Tablet (oral/sublingual), suppository, injection

anaesthetic. Other forms of local anaesthetic include local filtration, regional nerve blocks and epidural analgesia.

Table 7.3 lists analgesics and their form of administration for different levels of pain.

Frequently, more than one form of analgesic agent is required and the use of a sedative in conjunction with an analgesic has been shown to be effective. This is of particular relevance when undertaking painful procedures such as dressing changes. It may also be necessary for some patients to undergo repeated general anaesthesia for procedures such as dressing changes in order to minimise their pain

SUMMARY

In order to improve the management of pain in the burns patient, it is necessary to consider the following points.

1. Prevention is better than the cure.

2. Understand the importance of pain control.

3. Be aware of the physiology of pain.

4. Be aware of the various factors that affect the process of pain.

5. Do not rely on drugs alone.

6. Assess the patient for pain in an objective manner at regular intervals.

7. Promote patient involvement in the management of pain.

8. Encourage communication and co-operation between members of the multi-disciplinary team.

9. Be prepared to investigate the effectiveness of the wide variety of pain control methods that is available.

References

Crocker CG (1986) Acute postoperative pain: cause and control. *Orthopedic Nursing* **5**(2): 11–16.
Hayward J (1979) *Information: A Prescription Against Pain.* London: Royal College of Nursing.
Huskisson EE (1983) *Visual Analogue Scales.* In: Melzack R (ed.) *Pain Measurement and Assessment.* pp 33–370 New York: Raven Press.
International Association for the Study of Pain (1986) Classification of chronic pain. Descriptions of chronic pain syndromes and definitions of pain terms. *Pain (suppl. 3).*
McCaffery M (1979) *Nursing the Patient in Pain.* Lippincott Nursing Series. (Adapted for the UK by Sofaer B) London: Harper & Row.
McCaffery M and Beebe SA (1989) *Pain. Clinical Manual for Nursing Practice.* St Louis: Mosby.
Melzack R and Wall PD (1965) Pain mechanisms: a new theory. *Science* **150**: 971.
Sharpe S (1986) The use of the London Hospital Pain chart. *Nursing* **11**: 415–423.

Further reading

McCaffery M (1968) *Nursing Practice Theories Related to Cognition, Bodily Pain, and Non-environment Interactions.* Los Angeles: University of California.
Tortora GJ and Anagnoskos NP (1990) *Principles of Anatomy and Physiology*, 6th edn. New York: Harper Collins.
Watson JE and Royle JR (1987) *Medical-surgical Nursing and Related Physiology*, 3rd edn. London: Baillière Tindall.
Wolf ZR (1980) Pain theories: an overiew. *Topics in Clinical Nursing* **2**(1): 9–18.

8

Early Wound Excision

and Grafting

It is now acknowledged that early excision and grafting of the burn wound allows rapid wound healing, with a significant decrease in the incidence of wound infection, compared with a more conservative approach. However, experience is needed in selecting cases and the type of surgical excision.

Donor sites vary in thickness and healing rate. Dressings should be selected carefully, to suit the individual patient. They should also ensure that skin grafts are secured in place, as this is a very important factor in graft survival.

THE GENERAL PRINCIPLES OF EARLY EXCISION

Indications

Early burn wound excision is indicated in situations in which the wound will be slow to heal, i.e. taking longer than 2–3 weeks, which applies to deep partial thickness and full thickness burns. The procedure is used for larger wounds and also small deep burns in significant sites, such as the fingers.

Only superficial burns with bright pink wounds, demonstrating that a dermal circulation is present, and displaying wound sensation are obviously suitable for conservative treatment.

There are also other advantages of early surgery. Excision of the dead skin removes bacteria potentially harmful to the patient (Jackson and Stone, 1972), and early wound closure allows quicker recovery for the patient, with less pain, a reduced hospital stay (Muller and Herndon, 1994) and, hopefully, less scarring in the long term (Jackson and Stone, 1972).

Previously, a more conservative approach allowed the eschar (dead skin) to lift off gradually as a result of underlying bacterial action. This involved many dressings, pain and the need to graft on to granulation tissue (proud flesh) after approximately 2–3 weeks, with an increased chance of developing hypertrophic (thickened) scarring (Clarke, 1992a).

Early excision therefore helps to:

- Heal wounds more quickly
- Minimise infection
- Reduce the degree of scarring

Timing

Early excision, also called **tangential excision** ('shaving'), was first introduced by Janzekovic in 1969. Timing of surgery was between 3–5 days, when the burn wound had demarcated ('declared itself'). This is because progressive vascular changes are taking place in the first few days after the burn (Janzekovic, 1970). In the author's unit, we routinely check burn wounds at 48 hours post-injury and plan surgery, if needed, at that time.

Blood Loss

One of the acknowledged disadvantages of tangential excision is increased blood loss during surgery, Jackson and Stone, 1972; Heimbach and Engrav, 1984). This is anticipated, however, and there are ways of controlling blood loss, as well as limiting the amount of burn surface area treated. With major burns, it is safer to carry out a number of operations, with limited blood loss as a result.

Infection

Burns are, by their nature, enough to sterilise skin immediately following a thermal injury. Bacteria take some time to recolonise, and it is common for wounds swabs to show no growth for the first 3–5 days after injury. Most organisms will hopefully be shaved off, if present, during excision, but we routinely repeat wound swabs just before surgery to determine current flora. Immediate skin cover then protects the excised wound.

Antibiotic cover is given routinely, according to a set protocol, for 24 hours from induction of anaesthesia, to cover a possible bacteraemia (bacteria entering the blood stream) or septicaemia (growth of bacteria in the blood stream).

Healing

All skin grafts heal within 5 days, having survived for the first 3 days on a bed of serum. Cut capillaries gradually grow into the overlying skin graft – the process of inosculation (Jankauskas et al, 1991) producing a true capillary circulation. At 5 days, the graft should be pink, with a dermal circulation, and adherent to the wound bed, but will lack a nerve supply. (Skin grafts are not innervated tissue, although they may pick up some cutaneous nerve supply from adjacent nerves in due course.)

Scarring

Early grafting can produce very acceptable results despite the need to mesh skin grafts (Clarke, 1992a). The best results are obtained where the burn wound is deep dermal as opposed to full thickness. Despite shaving of the burn wound, some residual dermis is left underneath. This seems to maintain the skin's elasticity. Where there are breaches in the dermis down to the level of fat, skin grafts can then contract more readily, owing to lack of restraint from the missing dermis, resulting in hypertrophic scars. Pressure therapy is vitally important in helping to overcome this problem and also in the treatment of existing hypertrophic scars.

THE PROCESS OF SURGICAL EXCISION

Types of Surgical Excision

Tangential Excision

Tangential excision is also called 'shaving'. This implies that a surgical knife (with a guard) is preset, to allow dead skin to be removed (as in lathing wood) until bleeding dermis in the wound base is reached (Plate 1).

Fascial Excision

Fascial excision is carried out where the burns are deep, down to fat, with no chance of any viable dermis remaining. All skin and fat are therefore removed down to fascial level, usually overlying muscle. This is a vascular base, which readily accepts skin grafts. The procedure results in less blood loss, but there is a distinct disadvantage in that the contour is altered, resulting in a 'dip' or a 'wasted' appearance on, for example, a limb (Heimbach and Engrav, 1984) (Plate 2). This technique may, however, be the best means of providing rapid debridement (removal) of burnt tissue and wound healing, particularly in major burns, with enhanced survival as a result.

Blood Loss

Blood loss in burns surgery can be quite dramatic!

In order to be prepared for this, most patients need to have blood cross-matched before surgery, for example, up to as much as 10 units for a major burn. Surgeons should also help, by minimising blood loss during surgery; a number of procedures can be used to accomplish this.

1. Tourniquet on limbs – This makes surgery slightly more difficult. Experience is needed to ensure all the burned tissue has been removed, without taking off a layer of healthy tissue. Usually pink dermis and thrombosed vessels need to be removed – healthy dermis is pale white/yellow.

2. Diathermy – Cutting tissue with this technique cuts down blood loss. Also, coagulation diathermy (monopolar or bipolar) can be used for cut vessels.

3. Subcutaneous injection of adrenaline/hyalase solution – 1 ml 1/1000 adrenaline and 1 ampoule hyalase are diluted in 500 ml normal saline. This is then injected subcutaneously, under pressure, using a spinal needle. Blanching of the tissues results in a dramatic fall in blood loss from the burn wound and donor sites. Again, however, much experience is needed to gauge the correct depth of excision; slow capillary bleeding is considered to be the best guide (see below) and we find this particularly helpful for donor sites (Plate 3). Kahalley et al (1991) report a similar experience using a subcutaneous injection of a saline/vasopressor solution under donor sites and debrided areas with no problems in the healing of donor sites or skin grafts.

4. Topical agents – Epinephrine soaks are used in some centres (Heimbach and Engrav, 1984). Alternatively topical 5 vol-strength hydrogen peroxide (Cort and Herbert, 1971) may be used; this helps because of its exothermic reaction which coagulates the capillaries.

A more recent role of calcium alginate dressings has been their topical use as haemostatic agents on wounds, especially donor sites and excised burn wounds (NHS Surgical Dressings Information, 1988).

5. Skin It should not be forgotten that skin contains tissue thromboplastin, which initiates the 'clotting cascade' (Tortora and Anagnostakos, 1990). Hence, ready-prepared skin grafts are really one of the best means of controlling capillary bleeding.

Skin Cover

Prior to tangential or fascial excision, the first step should be harvesting (taking) skin grafts as this is the cleaner of the two procedures. Also, as mentioned above, application of skin grafts, already prepared, speedily stops oozing from the shaved wounds.

Skin can be meshed (except for the face) in a ratio of 1.5:1, to allow drainage to occur (Plate 4). This helps to prevent an underlying haematoma formation (collection of blood). The small splits in the grafts heal in 48 hours in a moist wound environment (James, 1992).

Cosmesis

Although meshed grafts (even minimally meshed 1.5:1) are not ideal, they can be fairly unobtrusive at 1–2 years and acceptable to patients. Some surgeons prefer non-meshed sheet grafts, even with tangential excision, but there is a risk of haematoma formation.

Hypertrophic Scarring

This is a frequent finding in burns scarring following more severe injuries (Plate 5). It is due in part to:

1. The depth of the burn – Deeper burns involving fat and a lack of dermis are more likely to develop thickened scars.

2. The site of the burn wound – It is more likely to occur on the chest, shoulders and neck area.

3. Racial factors – For example, West Indians may develop the worst form of hypertrophic scarring, known as keloid scars (Hugo, 1991).

4. Possible genetic causes – Hypertrophic scarring in Caucasians is more common especially in individuals with red hair.

SKIN GRAFTING

Split Skin Grafts

Thiersch Grafts

Karl Thiersch (1822–1895) was a German Army Surgeon in the Franco-Prussian War of 1870, who described the use of split-thickness skin grafts. The grafts are taken from a predetermined part of the body, using a skin knife, electric or air driven dermatome (Plate 6). Different thicknesses may be taken, depending on the need.

Meshed Grafts

Split skin is laid on a dermacarrier (mesher board) and fed through a skin mesher, which produces a series of splits, like a string vest (Plate 7). The main purpose is to allow drainage and prevent haematoma formation underneath. When there is a shortage of skin, however, the meshed skin can be pulled to widen the mesh (expansion), enabling it to cover larger areas.

Expansion ratios are 1.5:1, 3:1, 6:1 and 9:1, although there may be other combinations using other varieties of mesher. If the mesh is very wide, it is preferable to cover the skin with a biological dressing (e.g. specially prepared porcine skin) to protect the interstices. Again, this can be a life-saving procedure.

Any surplus skin grafts, either meshed or unmeshed, may be stored (clearly labelled) at 4°C in the skin refrigerator on the unit for up to 3 weeks and used for further grafting before being discarded. Alternatively, skin can be stored for a number of months using liquid nitrogen. Such a collection is described as a skin bank (Achauer, 1987).

Securing the Skin Graft

Remember the letter 'S':

- Superglue
- Staples
- Stitches
- Steristrips
- Simply vaseline gauze
- Splint
- Secure dressing

Remember also that skin grafts that lose their blood supply Slough off!

Wolfe Grafts

Julius Wolfe (1836–1902) was an Austrian ophthalmologist who later settled in Glasgow. In 1873, he described the repair of an eyelid using a postauricular graft.

Wolfe grafts are otherwise known as full thickness grafts. There is little place for them in the acute management of burns as they do not heal well in adverse conditions, i.e. possible infection and a potentially poor wound base. Also, donor sites are few. Split-skin grafts are more appropriate in the acute wound.

However, deep burns exposing tendon or bone require flap cover with skin containing underlying fat and its own blood supply. A Wolfe graft may rarely be used in this situation for the donor site, for example if a cross-finger flap has been used (Smith, 1990). Burns of this sort will not heal with a simple skin graft.

Hand burns benefit from moderately thick skin grafts to try to prevent the subsequent development of tight scarring. Also, some surgeons prefer sheet grafts to meshed grafts, but, as stated earlier, the risk of haematoma formation is higher as a result, and great care is needed at surgery.

Contracture Formation

The thinner the skin graft, the more it may contract. However, if the underlying dermis is partially present, this can prevent contraction, and a reasonable scar may result.

Where the dermis is virtually or totally lost the skin graft is liable to become thickened (compare an elastic band allowed to relax, having been stretched). This is especially likely to occur over fat.

Longitudinal bands of scarring may develop underneath, resulting in formal contracture bands (Plate 8) needing later release. This is necessary to protect in particular the joints from developing a diminished range of motion.

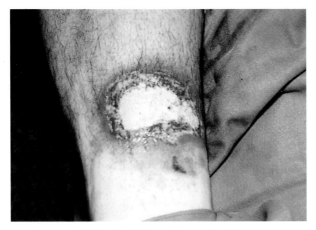

Plate 1. (a) Deep burn of calf.

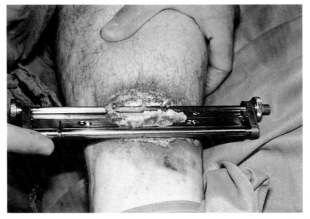

Plate 1. (b) Tangential excision (shaving) of deep burn of calf.

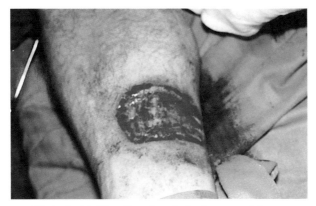

Plate 1. (c) Bleeding dermis in the wound base.

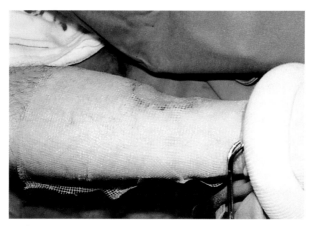

Plate 2. Wasted appearance following a fascial (deep) excision.

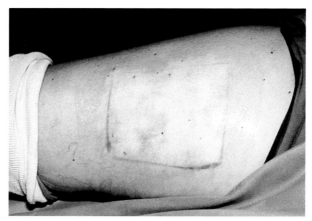

Plate 3. (a) Skin graft donor site injected subcutaneously with
adrenaline/hyalase solution producing blanching.

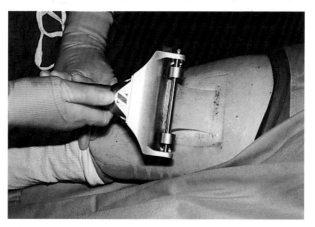

Plate 3. (b) Minimal blood loss during skin harvesting.

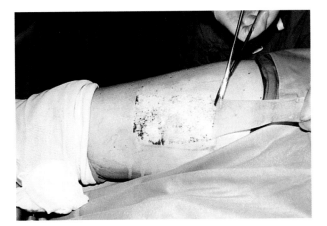

Plate 3. (c) Minimal capillary oozing from injected donor site following skin harvesting.

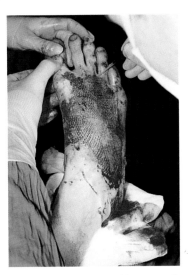

Plate 4. Meshed skin applied to a shaved burn on the foot, secured with Superglue™.

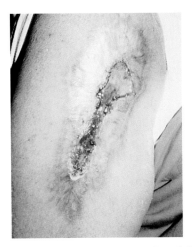

Plate 5. Hypertrophic scar developing in a burn of a right shoulder, not fully healed.

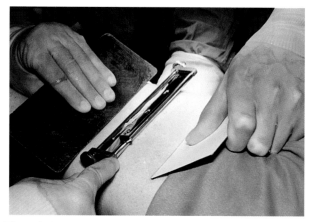

Plate 6. (a) Harvesting of skin using a Watson hand knife.

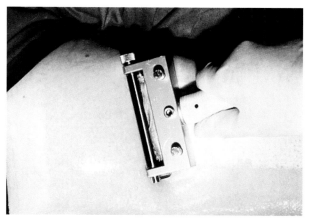

Plate 6. (b) Harvesting of skin using an electric dermatome.

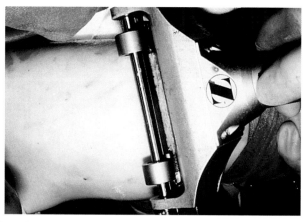

Plate 6. (c) Harvesting of skin using an air driven dermatome.

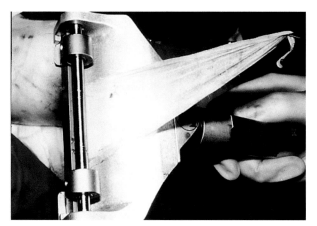

Plate 6. (d) The dermatome actually cutting a split thickness skin graft which may be taken of different thickness.

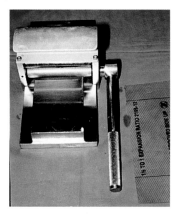

Plate 7. (a) Skin mesher and dermacarrier.

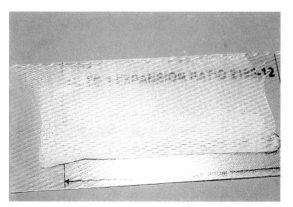

Plate 7. (b) Meshed skin spread on dermacarrier, meshed 1.5:1 (lower margin doubled over to obtain maximum benefit).

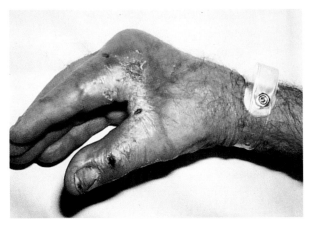

Plate 8. (a) Contracture of 1st web space of right hand.

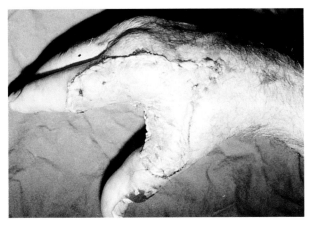

Plate 8. (b) Contracture released with insertion of thick skin graft.

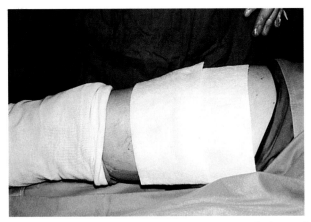

Plate 9. (a) Kaltostat dressing applied to skin graft donor site.

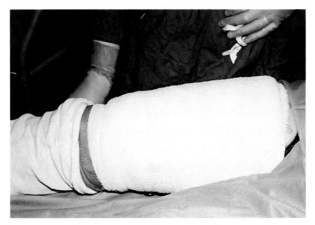

Plate 9. (b) Well padded donor site dressing.

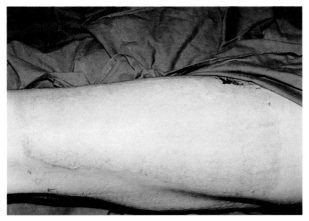

Plate 9. (c) Healed donor site after use of Kaltostat.

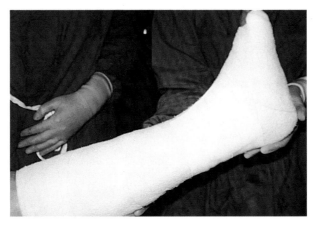

Plate 10. Splint applied following surgery to protect the skin graft.

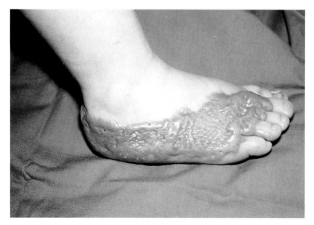

Plate 11. Active hypertrophic scarring.

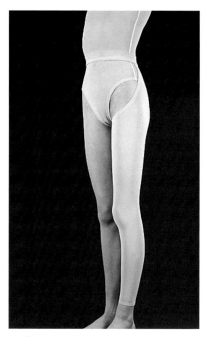

Plate 12. Lycra^{TM} pressure garments (courtesy of Camp Ltd).

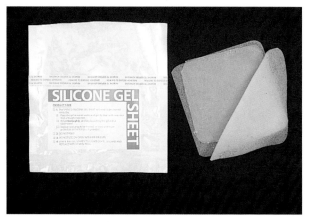

Plate 13. Silicone gel sheeting.

Cultured Skin

Cultured epidermal autografts (grown from the patient) have lost their popularity to a certain extent, owing to the need for laboratory facilities, the cost of production, the high failure rate and the quality of graft survival (Muller and Herndon, 1994). They are still used in major burns, however, where donor sites are scarce, and they can aid survival as a result.

BIOLOGICAL DRESSINGS

If skin graft donor sites are lacking in patients with major burns, temporary cover with cadaver or live donor skin (allografts) may be used. However, the individual must be appropriately screened to exclude viral transmission. Another alternative dressing is porcine skin (xenograft).

ARTIFICIAL SKIN

Artificial skin (Integra LifeScience Corporation, USA) has just been introduced into the UK and is an important new development in the wound management of major burns. It is a bilaminar membrane composed of a dermal portion of collagen and glycosaminoglycan (GAG), with an epidermal layer of synthetic silicone. The dermal portion serves as a template allowing infiltration of cells and neovascularisation. The patient's own collagen starts to grow as the dermal template disintegrates. Finally, the protective silicone layer is removed at about two weeks, to allow complete wound cover with thin split skin grafts from the patient.

THE PROCEDURE FOR OBTAINING A SKIN GRAFT FROM DONOR SITES

Donor Sites

Split-skin grafts can be taken from virtually anywhere in the body. However, places to avoid are the face, neck, hands, feet, perineum and breasts. This leaves the choice of:

- Limbs
- Buttocks
- Arms
- Abdomen
- Chest
- Scalp

For small grafts in children, the author's first choice is the buttock region, which heals well, despite any concern to the contrary. In adults, we prefer the inner thigh to the upper arm, which has been shown to be an area that may heal slowly, apart from causing an obvious cosmetic defect in females.

Skin thickness varies in different parts of the body (Tortora and Anagnostakos, 1990). The areas of thickest skin lie on the back and the sole of foot. The outer thigh skin is thicker than that of the inner thigh, an important point when looking for donor sites in elderly patients who have thinner skin. Care needs to be taken when harvesting skin in these patients: too thick a graft could result in a donor site not healing for many months, or even itself requiring a skin graft.

Lubrication

Friction is produced when shaving the skin off with a knife. Liquid paraffin wiped over the skin lubricates it satisfactorily; some surgeons also like to lubricate the knife. Care needs to be taken not to drip paraffin accidentally on the floor, causing someone to slip.

Equipment for Harvesting Skin Grafts

- Liquid paraffin – to lubricate the skin
- Skin knife/air driven dermatome – to cut the skin graft
- Skin boards – to steady or tense the skin
- Skin mesher – to mesh the skin graft
- Dermacarriers – to carry the grafts through the mesher
- Storage jar or tin – for storage of skin at 4°C for up to 3 weeks in a refrigerator

Blood Loss

Bleeding occurs from shaving or excision of the burn wound as well as from donor sites.

A recent paper estimated the total blood loss following surgery for adults to be 2.6%, and for children 3.4%, of their respective total blood volumes for each percentage burn excised or donor site harvested (Budny et al, 1993). We have found the adrenaline/hyalase subcutaneous infusion to be very helpful, resulting in much less blood loss. Blood transfusion and its attendant risks may be avoided as a consequence.

All swabs are weighed during surgery, to provide as accurate an account of blood loss as possible.

Reharvesting

It is possible to take skin from the same donor site, once healed, a number of times, in order to provide adequate skin cover (Cort and Herbert 1971; Clarke, 1992b).

Dressings

There are many dressings on the market (NHS Surgical Dressings Information, 1993) for donor sites. Different Burn Units may have individual preferences. Those dressings currently used the most are:

- Vaseline gauze
- Kaltostat
- Lyofoam
- Spyroflex
- Granuflex
- Opsite
- Omniderm
- Tegaderm

Healing Time

Children's donor sites tend to heal slightly more quickly than those of adults, at around 10 days as opposed to about 14 days. However, with the advent of calcium alginate (Kaltostat), healing times have shortened, and healing can occur as early as 5–7 days in some cases (Plate 9).

We avoid upper arms as much as possible now, following a Unit study, confirmed by others (Cort and Herbert, 1971), that showed adverse healing rates. If thick skin needs to be taken, it is possible to take a thinner graft from elsewhere to place on the donor site – this heals both areas more quickly (Press, 1991). Healing also depends on the patient's ability to heal and his nutritional status.

Cosmesis

Most donor sites heal very well with minimal scarring, and sensation is unaffected. Quite often the only evidence of injury is exaggeration of the hair follicles or less hair growth. Very occasionally, hypertrophic scars develop.

POST-OPERATIVE CARE OF THE WOUNDS

Dressings

If Vaseline gauze is used, it needs to be very well padded, to prevent 'strike through' (leakage of blood through the dressing). This must be treated quickly, to prevent bacteria entering the wound through the wet dressing; applying additional dry dressings may suffice. Otherwise, all the wet dressings down to Vaseline gauze may need to be removed and replaced.

However, Kaltostat needs fewer dressings due to its haemostatic properties and is now our standard choice of donor site dressing.

Exposure of the applied skin grafts may be carried out, if appropriate, on awkward areas in older children and adults, for example the buttocks, as this ensures a greater chance of graft survival. The grafts are observed at all times to prevent slippage, and blisters can be expressed.

Splintage is necessary to prevent grafts from shearing, if they are placed over or near joints that would otherwise move. This is usually achieved with plaster of Paris back-slabs or abduction splints (Plate 10). Occasionally, pre-formed splints are used, for example for abduction of the arms.

Removal of Dressings

Dressings should be left undisturbed, unless infection occurs. This is identified by pain, odour, seepage through the dressing or a raised temperature. The bandage must then be removed. If feasible, the patient is bathed, and if the donor sites are heavily infected, topical treatment with, for example, silver sulphadiazine cream may be necessary, as may systemic antibiotics if the patient is generally unwell.

Prevention of Deep Vein Thrombosis

All patients receive subcutaneous heparin (*Drug and Therapeutics Bulletin*, 1993) if they are on bed rest as a result of the burn or following surgery. Heparin is given twice or three times daily (if there have been previous problems), until the patient is fully mobile. Where practicable, anti-embolism stockings are also worn. Deep vein thrombosis can occur in burn patients despite the use of heparin therapy, and early detection is essential to prevent further complications.

Aftercare

Once the dressings are removed, the skin grafts and donor sites are very dry, owing to lack of sebum, which is normally produced by the sebaceous glands in the area (Janzekovic, 1970).

Moisturising with a bland cream up to five times a day is advised, to keep these areas supple. It may also help to reduce itching, a common complaint once the grafts and donor sites are healed, and it may especially help where the scars have become hypertrophic.

Sun Avoidance

Scars react badly following exposure to strong sun, exacerbating symptoms of irritation, redness and heat intolerance.

All burn patients need to avoid the sun and use total sunblock creams. Ideally, overseas holidays are better avoided the first summer after a significant burn – pressure garments anyway make swimming difficult! Holidays, should hopefully, be trouble-free, although may only become so for the burn patient 1–2 years after the injury.

References

Achauer BM (1987) *Management of the Burned Patient*, Ch. 6. University of California: Appleton & Lange.

Budny PG, Regan PJ and Roberts AHN (1993) The estimation of blood loss during burns surgery. *Burns – Journal of the International Society for Burn Injuries* **19**(2): 134–137.

Clarke JA (1992a) Late management of burns. *Surgery*, Plastic Surgery: 117–119.

Clarke JA (1992b) *A Colour Atlas of Burn Injuries*, Ch. 5. Roehampton: Chapman & Hall.

Cort DF and Herbert DC (1971) Practical aspects of skin grafting. *British Journal of Hospital Medicine* (Apr): 462–471.

Drug & Therapeutics Bulletin (1993) Preventing and treating deep vein thrombosis. *Drug & Therapeutics Bulletin* **30**(3): 9–12.

Heimbach DM and Engrav LH (1984) *Surgical Management of the Burned Wound*, chs 1, 2 and 4. University of Washington: Raven Press.

Hugo NE (1991) Hypertrophic scars and keloids. In: Smith JW and Aston SJ (eds) *Grabb & Smith's Plastic Surgery*, 4th edn, p 851. New York: Little, Brown.

Jackson DM and Stone PA (1972) Tangential excision and grafting of burns. *British Journal of Plastic Surgery* **25**: 416–426.

James MI (1992) The effect of synthetic dressings on wound contraction. MD thesis, University of Edinburgh.

Jankauskas S, Cohen K and Grabb WC (1991) Basic techniques of plastic surgery. In: Smith JW and Aston SJ (eds) *Grabb & Smith's Plastic Surgery*, 4th edn, pp 28. New York: Raven Press.

Janžekovič Z (1970) A new concept in the early excision and immediate grafting of burns. *Journal of Trauma* **10**(12): 1103–1108.

Kahalley L, Dimick AR and Gillespie RW (1991) Methods to diminish intraoperative blood loss. *Journal of Burn Care and Rehabilitation* **12**(2): 160–161.

Muller MJ and Herndon DN (1994) The challenge of burns. *Lancet* **343**: 216–220.

National Health Service (1988) Surgical Dressings Information. Welsh Common Services Authority National Health Service Pontypridd: Welsh Centre for the Qualioty control of Surgical Dressing.

National Health Service (1988) Welsh Common Services Authority Surgical Dressings information. Pontypridd: Welsh Centre for the Quality Control of Surgical Dressings.

Press B (1991) Thermal and electrical injuries. In: Smith JW and Aston SJ (eds) *Grabb & Smith's Plastic Surgery*, 4th edn, pp 706, 709. New York: Raven Press.

Smith PJ (1990) Skin loss and scar contractures. In: Burke FD, McGrouther DA and Smith PJ (eds) *Principles of Hand Surgery*, p 57. Derby / London: Churchill Livingstone.

Tortora GJ and Anagnostakos NP (1990) *Principles of Anatomy and Physiology*, 6th edn, chs 5 and 10. New York: Harper & Row.

9

Nutritional Care

in Burns Patients

Thermal injury places unique metabolic demands upon the body. Approximately 36–48 hours post-burn injury, following successful resuscitation from the shock ('ebb') phase, a severe catabolic state ('flow phase') develops. This is associated with significant weight loss, which can prove to be fatal. Nutritional support is vital to restrict weight loss and preserve lean body mass, thereby ensuring donor site and graft healing.

Nutritional support consists of three closely linked components: assessment of nutrient requirements, planning and implementation of dietary regimens, and monitoring the adequacy of the nutrients provided. This chapter discusses the theory behind current nutritional rationale and describes how this can be applied in practice.

Burn injury occurs more commonly in certain groups of the population than others. Those groups most at risk include young children, the elderly, and drug and alcohol abusers. Risk factors within these groups include poor economic and living circumstances within the family, such as limited cooking facilities, crowded housing and poor supervision of children, and the confusion or disabilities of patients who are mentally or physically compromised. These population groups tend to be at a greater nutritional risk and may already have been malnourished prior to thermal injury. It is important that these patients are assessed by a dietitian to determine their nutritional status, however minor the burn.

MINOR BURN INJURIES

Burn injuries of less than 15% body surface area (BSA) in adults and less than 10% BSA in children are classified as minor. In these, the basal metabolic rate (BMR) is not elevated to any great extent.

The BMR is the amount of energy that is needed to maintain physiological equilibrium while lying at rest in the fasted state. It represents a person's minimal daily energy requirement. Patients with minor burn injuries show an insignificant change in BMR, so that their nutritional requirements are similar to those requirements estimated for the general population (Department of Health, 1991). Body weight can usually be maintained through eating and drinking amounts similar to the patient's normal intake.

$$BMI = \frac{Weight\ (kg)}{Height\ (m^2)}$$

(measured in indoor clothing and without shoes)

Grades of obesity are defined as follows:

	BMI
Grade 0	20–24.9
Grade 1	25–29.9
Grade 2	30–39.9
Grade 3	>40

- Grade 0 indicates a desirable weight range
- a BMI of much less than 20 is suggestive of malnutrition
- Grade 3 indicates severe obesity

Fig 9.1   Body Mass Index

Both weight (kg) and height (cm) measurements are necessary if the dietitian is to determine whether a patient is over, under, or adequately nourished. Weight should be taken before dressings are applied.

These measurements should be calculated differently for adults and children. For children, growth charts should be used. When the measurements for weight and height fall on the same centile, this represents a child who is the ideal weight for his height. Children whose weight is more than a centile below that for their height suggests that they are underweight owing to an inadequate dietary intake. Extra attention should also be given to those children whose measurements fall on or below the third centile for both weight and height. The hospital admission is a valuable time for the dietitian to assess the adequacy of diet in such children and to educate the parents on appropriate feeding practices.

In adults, a formula called the Body Mass Index (BMI) is used (Figure 9.1). Particular attention should be paid to the dietary intake of patients with a BMI of less than 20. Use of oral supplements is likely to be necessary. Food intake should **not** be restricted in overweight patients while wound healing is being promoted.

MAJOR BURN INJURIES

The flow phase is characterised by an increased production of catabolic hormones (adrenaline, noradrenaline, glucagon and corticosteroids). These hormones cause

Intensive nutritional support is indicated if:

1. Burn > 30% total body surface area in adults
        > 25% total body surface area in children
        > 20% total body surface area in infants
   The range of values is due to differences in the surface area:volume
   ratio that exist between the different age groups.

2. The clinical course is likely to involve multiple operations; ventilatory
   support or compromised mental status.

3. For minor burns, the pre-burn nutritional status as assessed by
   growth charts or BMI and dietary/social history, is poor.

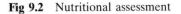

Fig 9.2   Nutritional assessment

a state of hypermetabolism, characterised by accelerated protein and fat breakdown, negative nitrogen balance and altered carbohydrate metabolism. The
abnormalities of carbohydrate metabolism include elevated blood glucose levels,
increased gluconeogenesis (glucose production from amino acids), altered insulin
levels and insulin resistance. If a patient also becomes septicaemic, this will further
accentuate glucose intolerance. Additional insulin should be given to treat hyperglycaemia. A reduction in carbohydrate and other nutrients is not appropriate and
would be detrimental to the patient.

   The hypermetabolic response is minimised by a warm environment, early closure
of burn wounds and prevention of wound sepsis. The burn size is a major consideration, as the metabolic rate increases in proportion to the size of the burn. Most
patients with a burn of greater than 20% BSA will exhibit an increase in metabolic rate.

NUTRITIONAL ASSESSMENT

Nutritional assessment should be carried out for all patients who may be nutritionally at risk (Figure 9.2).

   It is important to obtain a pre-burn weight in patients with major burns, as true
weight will become distorted through oedema, resuscitation fluid and bulky dressings. If this is not possible, the admittance weight minus that of resuscitation fluid
administered will be representative of the most accurate weight available.
Inaccurate weights may result in poor fluid and nutritional management. The
child's actual weight should be used if it falls on the 50th centile or above for age.
If the child's weight is less than this, the growth chart can be used to find the

weight corresponding to the 50th centile for age. This should be used instead of the actual weight to ensure the adequate provision of nutrients.

The literature on nutritional support for severe burns is based on adults, so extrapolation for children should be viewed with caution. Weight loss is expected in all patients. Dietitians aim to prevent a loss of more than 10% ideal body weight in adults. However, a loss of 10% ideal body weight in children is far more significant, as it represents a deviation in weight from the normal growth curve.

NUTRITIONAL REQUIREMENTS

Fluid Requirements

All fluid requirements in the first 48 hours are met through the standard fluid resuscitation procedure. Hence, any nutrition provided will be in addition to this. Following this period, requirements should be based on the recommended fluid intake (Department of Health, 1991; Elwyn, 1980) plus losses through evaporation. Evaporation losses are high in patients with large burns, owing to loss of the water-impermeable barrier. Wilmore and McDougal (1977) estimate fluid loss to be:

$$(25 + \% \text{ burn}) \times \text{body surface area (m}^2) = \text{ml water lost/hour}$$

This loss will reduce as the burn wounds heal.

Energy Requirements

Energy requirements are based on estimated energy expenditure. Total energy expenditure represents the sum of a number of factors including:

- Basal metabolic rate
- Resting energy expenditure
- Dietary-induced thermogenesis (DIT)
- Physical activity

DIT represents the energy expended during digestion and absorption of food.

Energy requirements can be calculated by direct or indirect calorimetry, or from a formula. Direct calorimetry involves calculation of heat production from a subject placed in a sealed chamber. This is impractical in the clinical setting.

Indirect calorimetry is becoming more widely used. A metabolic monitor may be situated at the patient's bedside and a canopy placed over the patient's head for between 20 and 30 minutes. This measures the amount of oxygen uptake and carbon dioxide produced. It provides a measure of the patient's resting energy expenditure (REE), i.e. the energy requirements at rest in the fasted state. Although this is the best method available for determining energy requirements, as it accounts for individual variability, it is expensive, complicated, time-consuming and labour-intensive.

Table 9.1 Equations for estimating energy requirements

1. Estimation of BMR (Schofield, 1985) + determination of energy requirements (Elia, 1982, 1990).

Age years	Male	Female
15–18	BMR* = 17.6 × wt† + 656	BMR = 13.3 × wt + 690
18–30	BMR = 15.0 × wt + 690	BMR = 14.8 × wt + 485
30–60	BMR = 11.4 × wt + 870	BMR = 8.1 × wt + 842
Over 60	BMR = 11.7 × wt + 585	BMR = 9.0 × wt + 656

*BMR is kcal/24 hrs. †Weight = wt(kg). The dietitian will adjust the BMR to account for stress, energy expenditure, DIT and pyrexia.

2. Elwyn (1980) provides some useful starting points for adults:

Change in BMR (%)	Nitrogen (g/kg)	Energy (kcal/kg)	Fluid (ml/kg)	Na (mmol/kg)	K (mmol/kg)
0–25	0.16	30	30–35	1.0	5.0
25–50	0.2–0.3	35–40	30–35	1.0	5.0
50–100	0.3–0.5	40–60	30–35	1.0	7.0

3. Energy requirements should not exceed twice the BMR.

4. Children: Dietary reference values for energy (Department of Health, 1991).

The most widely used method of calculating an individual's energy requirements uses formulae that are simple and incur no cost. However, there is no current consensus on the most appropriate formula to use, and a standard formula has yet to be developed.

Any of the proposed formulae have a reasonable expectation of accuracy in adults. The most frequently used formulae in the UK are represented in Table 9.1. Although many formulae over estimate requirements, the calculated intake is rarely achieved, owing to frequent interruptions related to nursing and surgical procedures. Days of underfeeding appear to have more clinical significance than those of overfeeding. There is substantial agreement that energy requirements plateau for burns of 50% body surface area and above, and energy expenditure rarely exceeds twice the predicted normal BMR. Many dietitians will compare the results of a few formulae to provide a baseline range of estimated energy requirements.

Recommended intakes for all nutrients have been calculated by the Department of Health (1991) and are known as dietary reference values (DRVs). Unlike the situation for adults, the normal recommended energy intake for a healthy child of the same age is often taken as the starting point, as the energy needs of children with major burns do not appear significantly to alter. It is suggested that hypermetabolism associated with major burns in children is compensated for by the large reduction in physical activity. However, it is important to remember that young infants and toddlers need to grow, so are particularly vulnerable to the effects of an inadequate diet. It is thought that growth will temporarily stop post-trauma. The energy normally used for growth can then be used in the healing process.

Energy requirements will need to be readjusted at 1–2 weekly intervals, in association with the reduction in hypermetabolism. The degree to which this occurs depends on the patient's weight change, the percentage wound healing, the presence or absence of infection and alterations in physical activity.

Protein Requirements

Protein requirements are known to be increased by severe burn trauma, because of increased protein turnover and protein losses through open wounds. It is not possible to prevent loss of body protein. However, the provision of protein at 2.5 g/kg ideal body weight for adults, which should represent approximately 20% of the total energy intake or twice the DRV for protein in children (3 g/kg ideal body weight for children under 12 kg), is sufficient to promote wound healing. Excessive protein may be detrimental to patients of all ages, and daily intake should not exceed 4 g/kg per day.

Growth hormone treatment in children accelerates donor site wound healing. Severely burned adolescents treated with growth hormone have shown greater protein synthesis than those not treated, increased protein synthesis contributing to more rapid keratinocyte replication (Muller and Herndon, 1994). However, growth hormone is extremely expensive and for this reason is rarely used in the UK.

Protein cannot be used without an adequate supply of energy. Therefore, nutritional requirements are often expressed as a non-protein energy:nitrogen(N) ratio, where 1 g nitrogen is equivalent to 6.25 g protein. In adult burn patients, this ratio is relatively low, owing to the large amount of protein required. It is suggested that a ratio (kcal/gN) in the range of 100:1 to 150:1 be provided.

Recent research has concentrated on specific nutrient manipulation to improve outcome. A number of different proteins have been tested, a few of which are discussed below (Paxton and Williamson, 1991).

Peptides (hydrolysed proteins) are more readily absorbed than are whole proteins or amino acids. They enhance sodium and water absorption, and may therefore play a useful role in the prevention or treatment of diarrhoea. It is also thought that peptides may improve nitrogen retention. Peptide-based complete enteral feeds are available, and may be the feed of choice in the early stages of treating critically burned patients.

Branched chain amino acids (BCAAs) have been suggested to stimulate protein synthesis and reduce muscle protein breakdown, but there is little current evidence to support this theory.

Glutamine is an amino acid that serves as a major fuel source for rapidly dividing cells, especially intestinal mucosal cells and lymphocytes. It is suggested that the addition of glutamine to feeds improves mucosal cell integrity and prevents bacterial translocation (see Early Feeding below). However, glutamine is unstable in aqueous solutions, so enteral feeds containing glutamine are in powder form, which has to be reconstituted with sterile water. Unfortunately, this increases the risk of contamination. It is current practice in some units to administer glutamine as frequent bolus feeds as part of the early feeding policy.

Arginine is an amino acid that is thought to stimulate the immune system by improving delayed hypersensitivity responses and clearance of bacteria. It also enhances wound collagen synthesis and decreases nitrogen loss. Arginine is stable in aqueous solutions and hence is available in a complete enteral ready-to-feed form.

Nucleic acids are the major structural units for DNA, RNA, ATP, etc. Rapidly growing tissues, such as intestinal epithelium and lymphoid cells, have a high requirement for DNA and RNA, and exogenous sources may be required during critical illness, owing to impaired synthesis by the liver. Addition of nucleic acids should improve and maintain cellular immunity and antibody production. Currently, there are few enteral feeds containing these proteins.

Carbohydrate and Fat Requirements

Carbohydrate and fat are both used to meet the non-protein energy requirements. Carbohydrate is a fuel for all cells and has a protein-sparing action by inhibiting gluconeogenesis. Excessive carbohydrate, however, increases hepatic fat deposition and carbon dioxide production, because of a limited capacity for glucose oxidation. The subsequent rise in respiratory effort associated with an increase in carbon dioxide production is of particular importance in the ventilated patient. Carbohydrate usually comprises 50–60% of the total energy intake.

Carbohydrate is provided as dextrose solutions (glucose source) for parenteral (intravenous) feeding, and as glucose polymers or maltodextrins in nutritionally complete enteral feeds and high calorie/high protein sip feeds.

Fibre (non-starch polysaccharides) is suggested to have an additional role in the treatment of critically ill patients, and is added to some nutritionally complete enteral feeds. Soluble fibre is broken down to short-chain fatty acids in the colon and may influence the integrity of the gut, thereby reducing the risk of bacterial translocation. Short-chain fatty acids also stimulate sodium and water absorption and may therefore be useful as an antidiarrhoeal agent (Paxton and Williamson, 1991).

As energy requirements are high and cannot be met through carbohydrate alone, fat is also used. This is a useful energy source and should provide approximately 20–30% of the total energy intake. Linoleic acid is an essential fatty acid and should be present in the feed to prevent essential fatty acid deficiency. Some of the total fat intake can be provided by medium-chain triglycerides (MCTs), which are readily absorbed and are rapidly available as an energy source (Paxton and Williamson, 1991).

Long-chain triglycerides fall into two categories depending on whether they contain omega-6 or omega-3 fatty acids. The former is suggested to compromise

Table 9.2   Vitamin and mineral requirements

Vitamin/mineral	UK DRV (adults)	Suggested supplement
Vitamin A	600–700 μg	5 ml Ketovite liquid or 0.6 ml Abidec
Vitamin B complex	B_1: 0.4 mg/1000 kcal	3 × Ketovite tablets or 0.6 ml Abidec
	B_2: 0.55 mg/1000 kcal	
	B_6: 1.2–1.4 mg	
Folate	200 μg	3 × Ketovite tablets
Vitamin C	40 mg	200 mg ascorbic acid or 0.6 ml Abidec
Iron	9–15 mg	200 mg $FeSO_4$ tablets b.d. or 2.5 ml b.d.–5 ml t.d.s. Sytron
Zinc	15–20 mg	220 mg $ZnSO_4$ or 5 ml $ZnSO_4$ mixture

Supplementation only applies if interal or parental feeding is not being used. The suggested supplements are of a common dosage, prophylactic in some cases, therapeutic in others, which aim to meet or exceed the DRV.

the immune system in large quantities, whereas omega-3 fatty acids, high concentrations of which are found in fish oils, may improve immunity. They have a possible role in the reduction of REE and catabolism (breakdown of body protein), improved protein synthesis and nitrogen balance, and better maintenance of overall patient weight.

Vitamin and Mineral Requirements

Specific vitamin and mineral requirements for patients with burns have not been established. Recommendations should be made by a dietitian on an individual basis, taking into account the pre-burn nutritional status and the amounts that will be supplied via sip and tube feeds. Care should be taken as it is possible to overdose the patient.

It can be assumed that requirements for certain vitamins and minerals will be increased, owing to their roles in metabolic pathways. The requirements for the B group vitamins will increase in proportion to the energy requirement, and the levels of most others should meet but not exceed twice their DRVs (Department of Health, 1991). Vitamin C should be supplemented in amounts up to 10 times the DRV, owing to its dominant role in wound healing. Additional iron should be provided if the patient is anaemic. Table 9.2 shows some of these vitamin and mineral requirements and suggested supplements, which exceed the DRV as detailed above. Commonly, Ketovite tablets and liquid® (Paines and Byrne) plus ascorbic acid tablets are given to adults, and Abidec® (Warner Lambert Ltd) is used in children. If anaemia is present, iron is given as iron sulphate tablets in adults or as Sytron® (Parke-Davis Medical) in children.

IMPLEMENTING DIETARY THERAPY

Calculated nutritional requirements are delivered via the enteral or parenteral route.

Enteral Feeding

Enteral nutrition consists of oral diets (plus supplements), nasogastric or nasojejunal feeding or feeding via a gastrostomy or jejunostomy, although the latter two routes are rarely used in burn patients. The enteral route is preferable for feed administration: it is simple, economical, safe and usually well tolerated. Enteral delivery is associated with preservation of intestinal integrity, including increased intestinal blood flow, reduced bowel oedema, improved gut motility and reduced rates of bacterial translocation (see Early Feeding below).

Enteral feeding (oral or tube feeding) should be started within 36–48 hours post-burn to minimise weight loss. Commencing within the first few hours post-burn, however, appears to be of greater benefit, owing to reduction of the hypermetabolic response (see Early Feeding below).

The dietitian will see and assess all patients identified as being at risk (see Nutritional Assessment above). Likes, dislikes, food intolerances and any other specific dietary requirements are identified. A dietary care plan is devised, comprising problems identified and aims and objectives of treatment. The nurse plays an important role in encouraging patient choice over food, ensuring that patients have ample time to eat and digest their meals. Treatments, procedures and other interruptions during meals should be avoided. Many patients will require assistance in eating. The nurse and dietitian will determine whether a normal diet is sufficient, and, if not, dietary supplements are offered in the form of high calorie/high protein sip feeds and/or the addition of a glucose polymer to fluids (Table 9.3). If nutritional requirements are not met orally within 2–3 days of commencing diet, some form of tube feeding should be used. Patients with major burns should automatically have a tube sited during the initial resuscitation period when the majority of invasive treatment is carried out.

Nasogastric (NG) feeding is still the most common form of tube feeding in the UK, although there is a risk of aspiration in patients who require supine immobilisation. The type of NG tube used depends upon the patient, body size and projected duration of feeding. Commonly, a wide bore tube, for example a Ryles tube of 12 French gauge (Fg) or more, is used in the intensive care unit, as it facilitates gastric aspiration. If the NG output is less than 600 ml per 24 hours, gastrointestinal tolerance is suggested. A wide-bore tube is uncomfortable for the patient as it is large and made from PVC, a fairly inflexible plastic, which may

Table 9.3 Oral supplements

Product	Description	Energy		Protein
		kcal/100 ml	kcal:Nitrogen	(g/100 ml)
0 years – adult				
● Polycal (C&G)	Glucose			
● Polycose (Ross Lab)	Polymer	100	–	–
● Maxijul (SHS)	Powders			
● Duocal powder (SHS)	CHO + fat	100	–	–
1–6 years				
Paediasure (Ross Lab)	Complete	100	183	3.0
Fortisip (C&G)	Complete	150	163	5.0
7 years – adult				
Build Up (Clintec)	Made up with whole milk	108	83	6.3
Ensure Plus (Ross Lab)	Complete	150	125	6.3

* A 1 kcal/ml solution is usually derived from:

10g (2 scoops [C&G]) glucose polymer
8g (2 scoops [SHS]) Duocal   } /100 ml milk or formula
25g (5 scoops [C&G]) glucose polymer/100 ml water or squash

inhibit a patient from taking fluids orally. Therefore, a fine-bore tube, preferably of 5–8 Fg (1–2 mm internal diameter), made of polyurethane or silicone, should replace it at the earliest possible moment. PVC tubes should be changed every 7–10 days, whereas tubes made of polyurethane/silicone can remain in situ for up to 6 months.

A 56 cm or thereabouts nasogastric tube should be used for children, and a 76 cm tube for adults. A 110 cm tube, weighted at the tip, is available for nasojejunal feeding. Nasojejunal feeding involves placing the tube by endoscopy beyond the pylorus so that patients with a gastric ileus can be fed safely. It is the most common form of feeding in the USA as it permits uninterrupted nutritional support during surgery, although the siting of these tubes places a high demand upon the endoscopy team.

Early Feeding

Early feeding, i.e. within the first few hours after a burn injury, is thought to be advantageous to the severely burned patient, even if only a small volume of feed is administered (McDonald et al, 1991). Without enteral feeding, changes in the gastrointestinal mucosal lining may facilitate the entrance of intestinal endotoxin and bacteria into the lymphatic circulation (bacterial translocation). This, in turn, stimulates the release of catabolic hormones responsible for the hypermetabolic state. Early feeding maintains intestinal integrity, thereby reducing bacterial

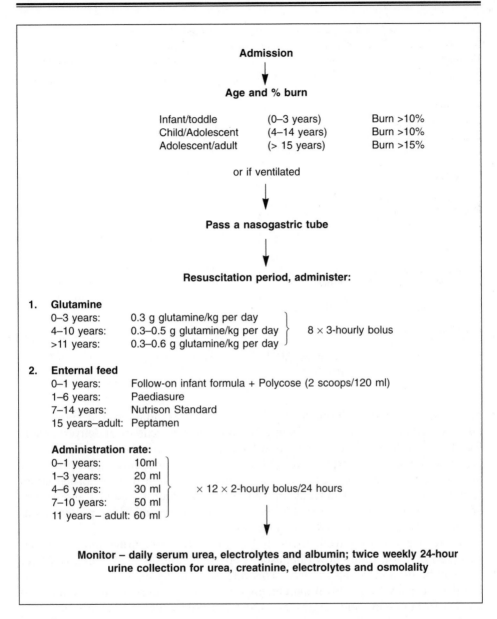

Admission

↓

Age and % burn

Infant/toddle	(0–3 years)	Burn >10%
Child/Adolescent	(4–14 years)	Burn >10%
Adolescent/adult	(> 15 years)	Burn >15%

or if ventilated

↓

Pass a nasogastric tube

↓

Resuscitation period, administer:

1. Glutamine

0–3 years:	0.3 g glutamine/kg per day	
4–10 years:	0.3–0.5 g glutamine/kg per day	} 8 × 3-hourly bolus
>11 years:	0.3–0.6 g glutamine/kg per day	

2. Enternal feed

0–1 years:	Follow-on infant formula + Polycose (2 scoops/120 ml)
1–6 years:	Paediasure
7–14 years:	Nutrison Standard
15 years–adult:	Peptamen

Administration rate:

0–1 years:	10ml
1–3 years:	20 ml
4–6 years:	30 ml } × 12 × 2-hourly bolus/24 hours
7–10 years:	50 ml
11 years – adult:	60 ml

↓

Monitor – daily serum urea, electrolytes and albumin; twice weekly 24-hour urine collection for urea, creatinine, electrolytes and osmolality

Fig 9.3 Suggested criteria for early feeding of the critically ill patient (first 48 hours)

translocation. It is also thought to prevent paralytic ileus. The benefits are not seen, however, if feeding is not instigated within the first 24 hours post-burn. Figure 9.3 represents a flow chart suitable for the early feeding of patients with major burns.

The dietitian will prescribe the most appropriate enteral feed for each individual and outline the method of administration, for example in terms of the pump

Table 9.4 Appropriate enteral feeds for burns

Product	Special features	Energy		Protein
		kcal/100 ml	kcal:Nitrogen	(g/100 ml)
0–1 years				
Follow-on formula + Duocal powder (SHS)		102	230	2.5
Pregestimil (MJ)	MCT, peptides	67	220	1.8
1–6 years				
Paediasure (Ross Lab)		100	183	3.0
Paediatric Nutrison (C&G)		100	223	2.7
7–14 years				
Osmolite (Ross Lab)		100	131	4.0
Jevity (Ross Lab)	Fibre	100	117	4.4
15 years–adult				
Fresubin 750MCT (Fresenius Lab)	MCT	150	100	7.5
Perative (Ross Lab)	Arginine, MCT, peptides	131	119	6.7

rate, time span and additions to the feed. Feed can be administered via gravity, but it is recommended to use a feeding pump to ensure accuracy of delivery. Table 9.4 illustrates the most commonly used feeds for burn patients and for which age group they are most appropriate. Follow-on formula are most appropriate for infants (under 1 year of age) as they are higher in protein than is normal infant formula. Normal paediatric feeds are suitable for children between 1 and 6 years of age, normal adult feeds for children aged 7–12 years, and high-protein feeds for adults and adolescents over 14 years of age.

The feed is usually introduced at full concentration but using small volumes, governed by a low pump flow rate, usually 30–50 ml/hour over 24 hours. A slower rate will be used in young children. This rate is gradually increased over the next 2–3 days, usually by 10–20 ml increments over 4–6-hour periods. Interruptions of feeding from nursing and surgical procedures, however, delays this process. Once established, tube feeding continues until the patient can consume sufficient nutrition orally. Invariably, 24-hour feeding changes to overnight feeding in an attempt to stimulate the patient's appetite during the day.

Poor tolerance of enteral feeding is indicated by vomiting, severe abdominal cramps and/or abdominal distension, worsening diarrhoea, or if the aspirated gastric content is greater than 50% of the volume administered during the previous 4-hour feeding period. The most frequent gastrointestinal complication is that of diarrhoea. This is often a result of antibiotic therapy, or, alternatively, the feed may be too hypertonic or the administration rate too rapid. Initially, the pump rate should be halved and the feed more gradually reintroduced. However, this compromises both fluid and nutrient intake, so should not be allowed to continue at a reduced rate for more than a couple of days. Alternatively, the feed can be changed for a less hypertonic one. Although diluting the feed results in dilution of all the nutrients, it is a useful way of meeting the fluid requirement. Once full volume is established, the feed concentration can then be increased.

Luminal obstruction of enteric feeding tubes is one of the most common mechanical complications. This can be caused by adherence of residue to tube walls or impaction of medications. Therefore, it is important to flush tubes with 20–50 ml sterile water, using a 50 ml syringe, before and after administering drugs and feed.

Parenteral Feeding

Total parenteral nutrition (TPN) is the aseptic delivery of nutritional substrates directly into the circulatory system, usually via a central venous catheter. It should involve a dedicated feeding line to reduce the risk of sepsis, and be administered via a volumetric infusion pump to ensure accurate delivery.

TPN proves to be an invaluable method of obtaining nutrition if the gut is inaccessible or not functioning. This is only likely to be necessary in patients with major burns who require ventilatory support in the Intensive Care Unit. However, it is the most expensive method of feeding and carries a high risk of sepsis. The hypermetabolic response seen in burned patients is not reduced by use of this route. TPN represents an unphysiological process associated with a greater risk of developing metabolic complications.

Peripheral parenteral nutrition (PPN) is not appropriate as the sole source of nutrition in patients with major burns because concentrated parenteral feeds, necessary to meet the high nutritional requirements, would cause phlebitis and occlusion of peripheral veins. It can be a useful adjunct to enteral feeding for those patients who are unable to achieve full nutrition via the enteral route alone, as it carries a lower risk of sepsis than does TPN and is easier to instigate.

The dietitian liaising with the medical team should determine the TPN prescription. The volume of TPN required is determined by the patient's calculated fluid requirements. There are two nutritional components of TPN: the water-soluble mixture, which is continually infused, and the lipid solution. The water-soluble mixture comprises carbohydrate, protein, electrolytes, minerals and water-soluble vitamins.

Carbohydrate is provided in the form of a hypertonic glucose solution, usually dextrose of 10%, 20% or 50% concentration. Dextrose should provide approximately 60% of the total non-protein energy intake. Occasionally, hyperglycaemia occurs. Insulin can be used to increase the clearance of glucose, but this is associated with increased fat deposition in the liver. Therefore, prior to administering insulin, a reduction in dextrose concentration without reducing the parenteral nutrition infusion will decrease the glucose load without compromising amino acid delivery. The lipid component can be increased accordingly to prevent a reduction in energy. If hyperglycaemia persists, however, insulin will be necessary.

Protein is provided in its most basic form (amino acids). These can be obtained from a product such as Vaminolact (Pharmacia Ltd) in infants, or differing concentrations of amino acid solutions in older children and adults. In adult burn patients, the more concentrated amino acid solutions are most commonly used, i.e. Vamin 18 (Pharmacia Ltd) or Aminoplex 24 (Geistlich Sons Ltd), providing 18 g and 24 g nitrogen/litre respectively, because of the high protein requirements. Electrolytes are added initially to meet normal requirements and then readjusted daily, depending on serum electrolyte levels. Vitamins and minerals are added to the mixture at standard recommended levels for intravenous nutrition. These are slightly lower than for oral requirements, as the gut is one of the regulatory organs that protects against trace element toxicity.

As discussed above, fat (lipid) is also a useful energy source and forms the second component of TPN. The fat solution, commonly Intralipid 30%, 20% and 10% Novum (Pharmacia Ltd) or Lipofundin 20% and 10% (B. Braun Medical Ltd) emulsions usually provide 40% of the non-protein energy intake. This should not exceed more than 60% of the total non-protein energy intake in adults 4 g/kg of lipid in infants or 2.5 g/kg of lipid in adolescents.

The lipid solution, together with fat-soluble vitamins, is commonly added to the water-soluble compartment to form a 'big bag' solution. These are mixed in pharmacy production units under strict aseptic conditions. Nowadays, it is preferable to use standard regimens available in ready-made bags, as this is much more cost-effective. However, these standard regimens are often unsuitable for patients with major burns as the non-protein energy:nitrogen ratio is too high.

TPN in infants may be made up daily by the pharmacy department. The water-soluble component should be given separately from the fat compartment. The latter, often only being a small amount, can be delivered via a syringe pump over 18 hours. This allows 6 hours for the lipid to clear from the blood prior to blood sampling, to ensure accurate results and check that the fat is being cleared from the blood. The concentration of divalent cations, for example Ca^{2+} and Mg^{2+}, is often too high in the young infant to allow mixing in one bag. Separate regimens allow for greater flexibility if alterations need to be made according to results from monitoring procedures.

Full-concentration TPN can be introduced in adults immediately. A flow rate of 1.5–1.6 ml/kg per hour is a good guide, depending on total fluid requirements. In infants and children, introduction is more cautious. The concentration of the regimen is usually increased over a few days, along with a gradual increase in the flow rate. The parenteral nutrition flow rate is normally increased by the same amount as the intravenous solution used to prevent dehydration is reduced. Full nutritional requirements are therefore not met for the first few days of TPN.

MONITORING

Monitoring is crucial to ensure that nutritional goals are being met. There is no single parameter that indicates nutritional adequacy. A combination of

Table 9.5 Format for completing food record charts

Time	Food offered	Amount eaten
8 a.m.	2 rashers streaky bacon	1 rasher
	2 large sausages	All
	1 grilled tomato	All
	2 slices thick white bread	1 slice
	with butter (thickly spread)	
	Tea with 28.5 ml full-cream milk	1 cup
	+ 1 tsp sugar	
10 a.m.	2 digestive biscuits	All
	Full-cream milk	200 ml
Noon	Fried fish in batter	Half-eaten
	Chips – average portion	All
	2 tbsp peas	1 tbsp
	1 portion jam sponge	All
	100 ml custard	80 ml
	30 ml undiluted orange squash	200 ml
	made up to 200 ml	
etc.		

measurements, such as nutrient intake, body weight, nitrogen balances and laboratory analyses, should be used and interpreted in the light of the clinical situation.

The nurse is responsible for administering the diet and monitoring the outcome. Oral intake (food and fluids, inclusive of sip feeds) is usually estimated by visual assessment and should be charted by nurses on a feeding form for all patients described as being nutritionally at risk. It is important to provide enough detail of the amounts eaten of each individual food or drink and the supplements taken (Table 9.5). The dietitian can use this information, plus the amount of intravenous or enteral feed delivered, to calculate the patient's actual nutrient intake and express it as a percentage of estimated requirements.

Body weight should be monitored weekly without dressings. Serial measurements can be compared to the pre-burn weight to calculate percentage weight loss. Weight loss should be no greater than 10% for patients with large burns, and preferably less than this in children.

Nitrogen balance is used as a measure of catabolism and helps to assess the adequacy of protein intake. It requires a complete 24-hour urine collection and accurate determination of protein intake. Nitrogen balance should be measured at least weekly. A simplified nitrogen balance calculation adapted from Lee and Hartley (1975) is commonly used by dietitians:

Nitrogen balance = Nitrogen input (g) – Nitrogen output (g)

Nitrogen output (g) = Urinary urea (mmol/24 hours) × 0.033

+ obligatory losses (hair, skin, faeces) of 2–4 gN

+ extra renal losses:

Pyrexia 0.6 gN/1°C
Burns exudate 0.2 gN/% BSA burn

The amount of burn exudate decreases as healing progresses. This occurs rapidly if the burn is of partial thickness. In full-thickness burns, exudate losses continue at 0.2 gN/% burn until the wound is grafted or the tissue has granulated. The burned surface area should be reassessed by nursing or medical staff at each dressing change, and the nurse should inform the dietitian of this. As the burn heals, nutritional requirements will alter. Metabolic rate and nitrogen losses peak at 5–12 days post-burn and lessen as healing and grafting occur.

Laboratory analyses for enteral feeding should include serum urea and electrolytes 2–3 times a week for the first 2 weeks, and then once a week. Blood glucose levels should be measured daily for the first 2 weeks. Liver function tests, full blood count and serum calcium, phosphorus and magnesium levels are required on a weekly basis. Weekly transferrin, albumin, mineral and trace element levels are also valuable. However, plasma proteins are poor predictors of nutritional status in the short term, owing to injury-induced changes. Transferrin has a shorter half-life (8 days) than albumin (20 days), so is a more sensitive measure. The trend in serial measurements of plasma proteins plays a more useful role.

Biochemical monitoring needs to be more aggressive when feeding parenterally, owing to the increased risk of complications. Laboratory analyses of urea and electrolytes, glucose and haemoglobin are required on a daily basis, and calcium, phosphate, albumin and transferrin levels and liver function tests should be recorded twice weekly until the patient appears to be clinically stable. The frequency can then be reduced to comply with the standard monitoring procedure for enterally fed patients. When introducing lipid parenterally as a separate component, lipidaemia should be tested for daily until the full dose of lipid is achieved. This cannot be done if a single-bag mixture is being used.

THE MULTIDISCIPLINARY TEAM

Good communication is essential if nutritional therapy of burned patients is to be effective. The medical team is responsible for biochemical monitoring and decisions on the stages of treatment. Nurses take the important role of assessing, feeding and monitoring their patients. It is obviously important to have good liaison with the catering department if a patient's needs are to be met within the constraints of a hospital environment. Pharmacists help in formulating TPN regimens and determining the most appropriate vitamin or mineral supplement. Occupational therapists help in ensuring that feeding is made possible through the use of specialised equipment. Play therapists can help young children by making eating fun, and psychologists can be invaluable through use of relaxation techniques and reducing patients' fears. Ward rounds provide a great opportunity to disseminate information from each of the professionals involved.

On discharge, patients who are of appropriate weight for height and who have been receiving a high level of nutritional support should reduce their intake to normal. However, if their food intake appears to be inappropriate, as observed by the nurse and dietitian, there is the opportunity for the dietitian and/or health visitor to educate the patient and family on healthy eating and how to achieve the dietary recommendations.

The use of any method of nutritional support requires careful administration and scheduled monitoring to ensure its safety and efficacy. Nurses have an integral role to play in assuring that appropriate nursing care and monitoring measures are performed.

References

Department of Health (1991) *Dietary Reference Values for Food, Energy and Nutrients for the United Kingdom*. Report on Health and Social Subjects no. 41. London: HMSO.

Elia M (1982) The effect of nitrogen and energy intake on the metabolism of normal, depleted and injured man. *Clinical Nutrition* **1:** 173–192.

Elia M (1990) Artificial nutritional support. *Medicine International* **82** (Oct): 3392–3396.

Elwyn DH (1980) Nutritional requirements of adult surgical patients. *Critical Care Medicine* **8:** 9–20.

Lee HA and Hartley TF (1975) A method for determining daily nitrogen requirements. *Post Graduate Medical Journal* **51:** 441–445.

McDonald WS, Sharp CW and Deitch EA (1991) Immediate enteral feeding in burn patients is safe and effective. *Annals of Surgery* **213:** 177–183.

Muller MJ and Herndon DN (1994) The challenge of burns. *Lancet* **342:** 217–218.

Paxton J and Williamson J (1991) Nutrient substrates – making choices in the 1990's. *Journal of Burn Care and Rehabilitation* **12(2):** 198–202.

Schofield WN (1985) Predicting basal metabolic rate, new standards and review of previous work. *Human Nutrition, Clinical Nutrition* **39C**, suppl 1(5): 41.

Wilmore DW and McDougal WS (1977) Nutrition in burns. In Richards JR and Kinney JM (eds) *Nutritional Aspects of Care in the Critically Ill*, pp 583–594. Edinburgh: Churchill Livingstone.

10
Rehabilitation

The 'team' approach to the management of a burn-injured patient is essential, and the physiotherapist has an important role to play in the patient's rehabilitation. The roles of individual members of the multidisciplinary team will naturally overlap, and the nurses, physiotherapist and occupational therapist will need to work closely together (Bach et al, 1984). Good communication between each member of the team is essential so that everyone works together towards agreed goals.

The ultimate aim is for the patient to return to full independence, managing his or her former occupation and hobbies wherever possible.

The *aims of physiotherapy treatment* are to:

- Maintain clear airways
- Prevent joint contracture
- Aid functional independence
- Provide psychological support

MAINTENANCE OF CLEAR AIRWAYS

Smoke Inhalation

A smoke inhalation injury may be diagnosed if the patient has been trapped in a smoke-filled room and has facial burns, singed nasal hairs, soot in the mouth, impaired voice and signs of respiratory distress (Mathur, 1986). Smoke consists of heat, gases and particulate matter (Kinsella, 1988). The main gaseous content comprises oxygen, carbon dioxide, carbon monoxide and hydrogen cyanide. Oxygen is consumed in the process of combustion, and inhalation of carbon monoxide will further reduce the available oxygen to the tissues, resulting in the patient becoming hypoxic. Cyanide poisons the mitochondria and affects cellular metabolism, which will aggravate the metabolic acidosis caused by hypoxia (Kinsella, 1988). The heat from smoke particles can cause thermal damage when deposited in lower airways, and the smoke particles can directly cause airway irritation. Inhalation of smoke may also cause bronchospasm, pulmonary oedema and the production of sooty sputum. The patient is therefore at risk of developing a chest infection.

Patients with a smoke inhalation injury often have accompanying burns to the face, which can become grossly swollen in the first few days. The eyes can become so swollen that the patient cannot see, so it is particularly important that the physiotherapist explains all procedures to the patient. To allow gravity to help the facial oedema to drain, patients are usually nursed upright, but they may have to be repositioned during physiotherapy treatment to aid drainage of sputum. Deep breathing exercises are encouraged, and, by vibrating or percussing the patient's chest, the physiotherapist aims to loosen any secretions. The patient is then encouraged to cough and expectorate, so that the lungs are kept clear.

If the patient has bronchospasm, the administration of a bronchodilator via a nebuliser prior to chest physiotherapy may also help to loosen secretions.

In severe cases of smoke inhalation, endotracheal intubation may be necessary to prevent occlusion of the airway owing to oedema (Mathur, 1986). The patient may also need to be ventilated and monitored in the Intensive Care Unit. Once ventilated, the patient cannot usually clear his own sputum, and regular chest physiotherapy and endotracheal suction may be necessary.

Other Causes of Retained Secretions

Patients who have a past history of chest problems, for example asthma and bronchitis, may be more at risk of developing a chest infection. This is particularly so if they are elderly, are having repeated general anaesthetics, and are confined to bed to allow skin grafts to heal. The physiotherapist will teach the patient breathing exercises and how to clear any secretions, and encourage early ambulation whenever possible.

PREVENTION OF JOINT CONTRACTURE

Exercise

Any joint whose overlying skin has been damaged by a burn has the potential to become stiff and eventually contracted if the joint is not regularly exercised. It is always better to prevent a joint contracture from occurring than to treat it (Boswick, 1983).

For the first 48 hours, most areas are heavily bandaged, making exercise very difficult. The first occasion for the physiotherapist to assess and encourage joint movement is when all the dressings are removed, 48 hours post-injury, for the depth of the burn to be assessed by the medical staff (Gairns and Martin, 1990). The physiotherapist will then encourage the patient to move each affected joint through as full a range of movement as possible. Another good time for the physiotherapist to encourage the patient to exercise his joints is when the patient is in the bath (Giuliani and Perry, 1985; Raeside, 1992). Again, dressings do not impede movement, and it is often easier for patients to move their limbs in a relaxing warm bath. Treatment sessions will, in this instance, have to be kept brief so that the patient does not get cold.

Good pain control is essential so that the patient can achieve an optimum range of movement in each joint (Raeside, 1992). The physiotherapist will endeavour to time treatment with the administration of analgesia. If oral analgesia is not effective and circumstances permit, the physiotherapist may administer entonox during treatment.

Hand burns are worthy of a special mention. Finger joints are very sensitive and can stiffen very quickly. The hand can also become grossly oedematous, which similarly prevents joint movement (Carmudie, 1980). It is therefore imperative that the hand is kept elevated in a Bradford sling (Figure 10.3) at all times to allow the oedema to drain. It is also essential that dressings to the hand are as light as possible, so that the patient can regularly exercise on his own. The use of plastic or semipermeable membrane bags are ideal as they allow free movement of the fingers (Gairns and Martin 1990; Martin et al, 1990). Therefore, regular exercise of affected joints is encouraged as soon as possible after the patient is admitted.

If the patient has to have skin grafts, exercises are stopped for 5–7 days to allow the grafts to heal (Carmudie, 1980). Once the doctor is happy that the skin grafts are stable, exercises can be resumed. Initially, this is best carried out with the dressings off so that the physiotherapist can observe the grafts. Again, in post-grafted hand burns, it is imperative that the dressings are as light as possible so that the patient can be encouraged to exercise and use his hands.

Most young children do not require physiotherapy treatment as their joints do not stiffen as quickly as those of adults. If exercise is necessary, the physiotherapist may need to use his or her imagination in devising play activities to encourage movement at the required joints (Raeside, 1992). The assistance of the nursery nurse can be of great benefit in these circumstances.

Positioning

The position that the patient is resting and sleeping in needs to be monitored to control oedema and to help prevent joint and skin contractures from developing (Boswick, 1983). As a general rule, the position of contracture for most joints is flexion. This means that the patient should not be spending any length of time with a joint in a flexed position if it has overlying skin grafts. The patient needs to be encouraged to keep the joint in a position opposite to that of contracture (Boswick, 1983). Hence patients should not have pillows under their knees if the flexor aspect of the knee has been grafted (Figure 10.1), or more than one flat pillow under their head if the flexor aspect of the neck has been grafted (Figure 10.2). Hand burns need to be elevated (Figure 10.3), and patients with facial burns should sit upright to help to control oedema. To help prevent a contracture following burns to the axilla, the patient's arm may have to be positioned in abduction on several pillows or on a bed table (Figure 10.4). The patient may also need to sleep in this position, and encouragement by the nursing staff as well as the

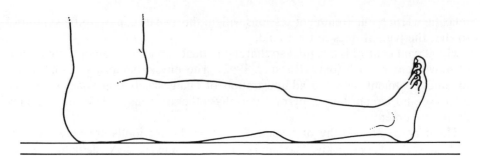

Fig 10.1   Resting position for leg burns

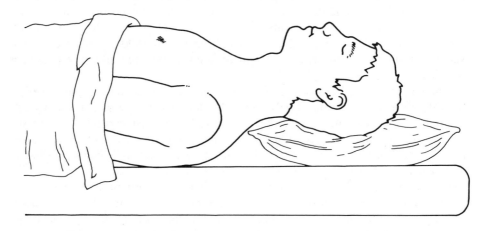

Fig 10.2   Resting position for anterior hand burns

physiotherapist will help to reinforce this. A patient who has had burns to the
flexor aspect of the hip may need to spend some part of each day in the prone
lying position (Figure 10.5) to help prevent a flexion contracture at the hip.

Splinting

If exercise and positioning are not sufficient in maintaining a joint in correct align-
ment, a splint may be required. This is particularly important in patients with
hand burns who are ventilated and sedated and are therefore unable to cooperate
with hand exercises. The hands are splinted in a position that will help to prevent
joint contractures: the wrist in slight extension, the metacarpophalangeal joints
in flexion, the proximal interphalangeal joints in extension and the thumb in
abduction (Bach et al, 1984) (Figure 10.6). The splints are worn at all times, only
being removed for change of dressings and twice daily by the physiotherapist so
that a full range of passive movement to the fingers, thumb and wrist can be
carried out.

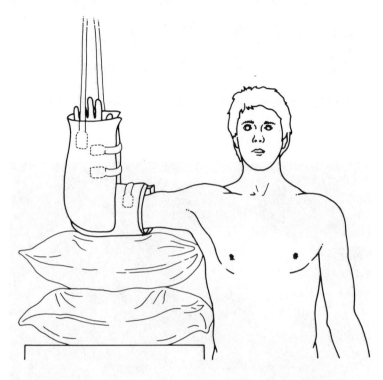

Fig 10.3   Resting position for hand burns, also illustrating a 'Bradford' sling

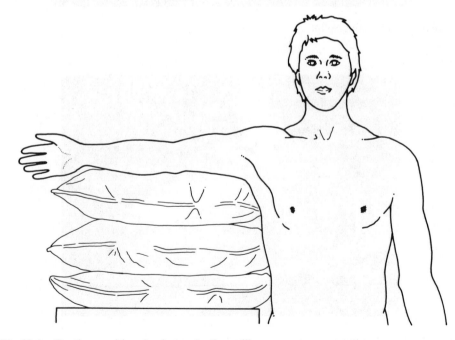

Fig 10.4   Resting position for burns to the axilla

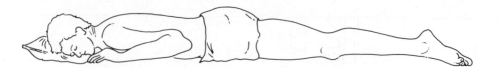

Fig 10.5   Position for a patient with burns to the flexor aspect of the hips

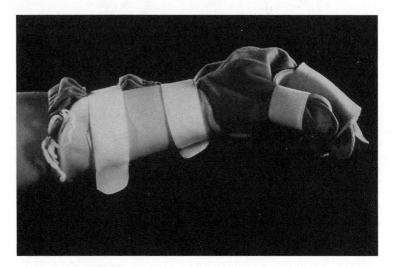

Fig 10.6   Hand resting splint

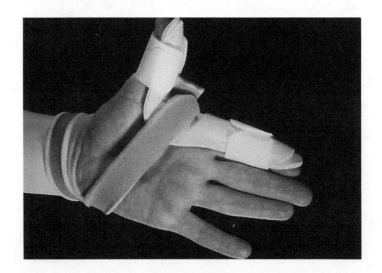

Fig 10.7   Thumb abduction splint for burns to thumb web

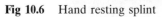

The physiotherapist or occupational therapist will usually make a splint from a thermoplastic material, which is heated in hot water to soften it (Carmudie, 1980). When sufficiently cool, it is moulded over the patient's dressings to hold the joint in a corrected position. The splint material becomes virtually rigid once it is completely cool.

Splints may be worn day and night, only being removed for exercise or change of dressings, or they may be worn just at night, the patient being left free to exercise regularly during the day. The splint can be held in place by a bandage or by Velcro straps (Figures 10.7, 10.8 and 10.9).

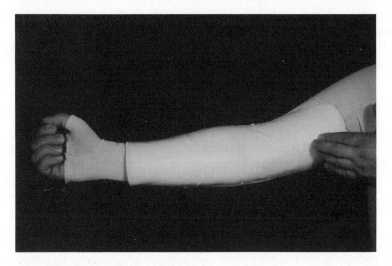

Fig 10.8   Elbow extension splint

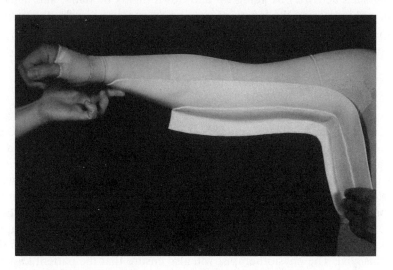

Fig 10.9   Arm abduction splint

AIDING FUNCTIONAL INDEPENDENCE

Ambulation

Patients with leg burns are encouraged to mobilise as soon as possible. Skin grafts to the lower limbs need to be supported by correctly sized, double-thickness tubigrip, which will help to control oedema and prevent venous stasis (Giuliani and Perry, 1985). The physiotherapist may need to provide a suitable walking aid, such as a walking frame, crutches or a stick. Close liaison with the nursing staff is essential so that the patient can be encouraged to walk to the bathroom or toilet when the physiotherapist is not present. The physiotherapist may also have to teach the patient how to negotiate stairs and ensure that he is safe before discharge home is considered.

Exercise Tolerance and Muscle Power

Patients who have had frequent visits to the operating theatre, resulting in periods of time on bed rest, very quickly become weak and debilitated (Giuliani and Perry, 1985). The physiotherapist will encourage patients to increase their exercise tolerance by taking them on longer walks, perhaps also visiting the physiotherapy department for activities in the gym. This also takes the patient out of the protected environment of the Burns Unit and helps him to prepare for a return to normal society.

If the patient is confined to his room because of a wound infection, he may benefit from using a static bicycle, which can be kept in the room. By gradually increasing such activities as going up and down flights of stairs, and activities in the gym, and increasing the length of time on an exercise bicycle, the patient will gradually increase his muscle power and strength (Boswick, 1983).

Self-care and Independence

As a preparation for discharge home, the patient is encouraged to be as independent as possible in all daily activities (Giuliani and Perry, 1985). If the patient has injured hands, the physiotherapist will check that he is using his hands for functional activities as well as continuing with regular exercise. The patient needs to be as independent as possible, particularly if living alone. The patient will have to be able to put moisturising cream on grafted areas, be independent in getting in and out of a chair and on and off the bed or toilet, and negotiate the stairs safely before discharge from hospital can be arranged. The physiotherapist will therefore need to work closely with the patient and other members of staff to achieve this goal. The physiotherapist will also ensure that the patient knows what exercises to continue doing at home.

PSYCHOLOGICAL SUPPORT

Most burn-injured patients have difficulty in coming to terms with their injuries and can go through various stages of anxiety, depression or even aggression (Giuliani and Perry, 1985). The physiotherapist has an ideal opportunity to establish a relationship with the patient during treatment sessions and will be able to offer support and encouragement when necessary. Parents of a burn-injured child may need to supervise exercises or appropriate play activities when their child returns home (Raeside, 1992). The parents may need help and support at this time, particularly if the child is unwilling to co-operate. Patients may have many questions and anxieties about scarring, altered body image and how they will manage at home or at work, and these anxieties may be voiced to the physiotherapist during treatment sessions. When appropriate, the physiotherapist will be able to offer reassurance and advice.

OUTPATIENT FOLLOW-UP

After discharge from the Burns Unit, the patient may need to continue with physiotherapy treatment as an outpatient (Raeside, 1992). The physiotherapist will normally review the patient when he attends for a change of dressings, as it is usually easier to monitor joint movement when the dressings are removed. Hand burns, in particular, may need monitoring for some time to ensure any graft tightness does not result in joint contracture. Splintage may also need to be considered at this stage.

Younger patients who are keen to regain their former fitness and strength may benefit from intensive physiotherapy and occupational therapy at a rehabilitation centre. This can serve as a good preparation for the patient to return to work.

CONCLUSION

The physiotherapist has an important and often demanding role in the rehabilitation of a burn-injured patient, requiring patience, adaptability and often a firm but caring approach. The ability to work with other members of the multidisciplinary team is essential, and it is close team work with patients that will help them to overcome their injuries.

References

Bach J, Draslov B and Jørgensen B. (1984) Positioning, splinting and pressure management of the burned hand. *Scandinavian Journal of Plastic and Reconstructive Surgery* **18:** 145–147.
Boswick JA (1983) Rehabilitation after burn injury. *Annals of the Academy of Medicine* **12**(3): 443–448.

Carmudie C (1980) Management of the burned hand. *Australian Journal of Physiotherapy* **26:** 4.

Gairns CE and Martin DL (1990) The use of semi-permeable membrane bags as hand burn dressings. *Physiotherapy* **76**(6): 351–352.

Giuliani CA and Perry GA (1985) Factors to consider in rehabilitation aspect of burn care. *Physical Therapy* **66**(5): 619–623.

Kinsella J (1988) Smoke inhalation. *Burns* **14**(4): 269–279.

Martin DL, French G and Theakstone J (1990) The use of semi-permeable membranes for wound management. *British Journal of Plastic Surgery* **43:** 55–60.

Mathur NK (1986) Inhalation injury in major burns. *Care of the Critically Ill* **2**(5): 195–196.

Raeside F (1992) Physiotherapy management of burned children: a pilot study. *Physiotherapy* **78**(12): 891–895.

Further Reading

Leveridge A (1991) *Therapy for the Burn Patient.* London: Chapman & Hall.

11

Social Reintegration of the Burn Patient

When admission to the Burns Unit takes place, the most common question asked by families and the patient is 'How long will the patient be in hospital?' This immediate concern is acknowledged by the burns nursing team, and therefore, irrespective of the severity of the burn injuries, the Nottingham Burns Unit has developed a social reintegration programme, which begins on admission and continues in stages, until long-term rehabilitation for both patient and family has successfully taken place.

STAGE 1: SOCIAL ISOLATION/FAMILY INVOLVEMENT

After assessing the burn injuries, an experienced specialised burns nurse, i.e. the named nurse (Department of Health, 1991), will then be able to determine the extent to which the social reintegration programme is needed.

Many factors will influence patients' responses to their physical injuries, depending on their age, the situation surrounding the burn incident and the location or severity of burn, for example of the face or with regard to the percentage of body surface area burnt. The primary nurse (known as the keyworker) will consider all these reactions when planning and providing the holistic care for the patient, in order to maximise psychosocial recovery.

Isolation

Isolation, whether protective or social, is a very traumatic and stressful experience. It is usually experienced in the acute phase of care and/or if an infection has invaded the burn wounds. Marvin and Seligman (1991) suggest that there may be numerous reasons for the patient's feelings of isolation:

- Alterations in appearance
- Loss of previous role functions in life
- Loss of or impaired sensory motor functions
- Alterations in interpersonal relations as the result of being hospitalised

It is therefore important for the keyworker to understand and be aware of any signs and symptoms that would relate to isolation and psychosocial readjustments.

A patient may sometimes withdraw from social interactions and/or interactions with the family. This is often their only means of coping. Feelings of hostility and anger may also be present. These feelings or psychosocial responses are usually complicated by further defence mechanisms, depending on the developmental differences in the patient:

1. *Regression*, which is seen mostly in children, is usually a way of dealing with stress i.e. fear, anger, loneliness and pain (Campbell, 1976). The patient reverts to an earlier stage of development which enables him/her to cope by, for example:

- *refusing to take food and fluids* – this power struggle, between nurse or parent and child leads to unco-operative behaviour
- *wetting the bed and defaecating* – the child lets go control of the bladder and bowel, in order to vent anger and frustration.

2. *Repression*, which is more likely to be an adult's response to coping, is described by Mendelssohn (1984) as an 'automatic barring from consciousness of anxiety producing thoughts or feelings'. An example of this is the common response of refusing to talk about the future, or sometimes the inability to acknowledge or even look at the burn injuries. This denial shows an inability to cope.

The keyworker, aware of these potential problems, should provide a plan of care that is individualised for particular needs, i.e. maintaining the patient's independence, encouraging social interactions with the family and friends, and minimising the patient's pain and discomfort.

Communication skills and trust need to be established and developed as rapidly as possible by the nurse. Partridge (1991) explains that this will give feelings of comfort and security to the patient, which in turn boosts the patient's morale.

Family Involvement

Family members are encouraged to be involved in all aspects of active and psychosocial care, as much as they are willing and able to. This can be difficult at first, as many factors may influence their behaviour:

- Role change
- Anxiety and shock
- Lack of confidence
- Lack of support from other members of family
- Guilt

Families therefore need to be supported by the keyworker and the burns team. Identifying the needs of the family, and establishing a rapport between nurse and family, should hopefully alleviate some of the above factors, and, in time, the relationship that evolves between patient, family and nurse will promote trust and confidence.

Family involvement has two aims, to establish:

1. A feeling of comfort and security for the patient
2. A feeling of usefulness, control and self-worth for the family

With these two aims in mind, the Burns Unit provides facilities for the family to be resident within the unit. Families are encouraged to bring in personal belongings and effects, which will enhance the comfort of the patient while he is socially isolated; such items may be photographs of family and pets, familiar objects, music tapes, videos, pictures and toys, and as well as favourite foods and drinks.

The keyworker should express to the family that showing the patient their love and concern will both reassure the patient and give comfort to themselves. The importance of touch, as suggested by Manger and Speed (1986) should also be emphasised. Stroking the uninjured skin, holding or cuddling the patient and sharing a kiss will alleviate the patient's feeling of isolation.

STAGE 2: SOCIAL INTERACTIONS (ADULTS/CHILDREN)

As the patient begins to heal from the injuries, social interactions and activities will be encouraged. Departmental visits, for example to the gymnasium and Occupational Therapy Unit, within the hospital will usually be the first step out of the Burns Unit. These visits will help the patient to develop confidence by meeting familiar people in new surroundings.

Once these have been established, the patient can then progress to other areas within the hospital, for example the cafeteria and social club. This can be difficult in the beginning, with the stares of others and unsightly scars on limbs, but with persistence and time, coping strategies will hopefully overcome fear and self-consciousness.

When the patient and the family feel confident enough, small social activities, such as walking around the grounds of the hospital or visiting a local cinema, park or shops, are encouraged.

After returning to the Burns Unit, patients are given time to discuss and express their feelings about the 'outing': How did they feel? Did they have any problems?

After establishing that the patient is able to cope with the outside environment, Stage 3 can begin.

Play and Education (Children)

Play is essential for the child who has burn injuries. Douglas (1993) describes how it helps to resolve stressful situations, reduces anxieties, facilitates communication and speeds recovery and rehabilitation.

On admission to the Burns Unit, the child's room is made to appear as non-clinical as possible. Appropriate to the age of the child, books, toys and videos are placed in the room. Hospital bedding is disguised with colourful cartoon bed coverings. These distractions provide some comfort to the child and alleviate initial fear.

The child and family are introduced to the full-time nursery nurse (who is employed on the Burns Unit) as soon as possible after admission. Her role is to find out what activities the child/adolescent takes part in at home and to incorporate these into care. The nursery nurse will attempt to stimulate the child or adolescent with interests, for example computer games and drawing, that will keep him occupied and will progressively help with mobility of post-burn limbs at a later stage of rehabilitation.

The nursery nurse also provides extra emotional support for the child in the absence of the parents.

Once the child's wounds have begun to heal, he will be encouraged to become a little more independent. If possible, he will move into the children's ward area containing four beds, in order to be stimulated by other children and take part in play activities.

A playroom in the Burns Unit is provided for infants and preschool children. This is a 'safe' environment for children where no clinical procedures are undertaken.

For the school-age child, there is a need for play and educational activities. When the child is well enough, a hospital teacher will be arranged to facilitate the educational needs of the child. Adolescents must be given the opportunity to continue with school work in a suitable environment, so that on discharge they will be able to reintegrate quickly.

STAGE 3: VISITS HOME

As the burns patient begins to recover, it is possible to begin the preparation for discharge. Between the keyworker, patient and family, discussions will take place to ensure a smooth, progressive step into going home. Depending on how far away the family lives, this usually begins with a day out visiting home. The patient is able again to familiarise himself with his home surroundings and renew social bonds with immediate family and friends.

This can be a very emotional and sometimes distressing experience, especially · if the burn incident happened at home. The family need to give their loved one time to express feelings and emotions while at home, as well as giving reassurance, so that the individual can develop coping mechanisms.

On return to the unit, more discussions will take place between the keyworker, patient and the family to ensure that there were no physical or psychological problems that may need to be solved before discharge.

STAGE 4: WEEKEND VISITS

The weekend visit home deliberately includes provision of some physical care, which is not supervised. This gives the family a chance to develop their own abilities and confidence for the individual's permanent return home. As before, discussion on how successful the visit was will take place on return to the Burns Unit.

STAGE 5: DISCHARGE

Discharge from the Burns Unit to home is a very emotional experience. It is a period of adjustment for both patient and family. It is therefore important that support and a flexible approach to providing help is led by the keyworker, who cares for the patient and the family throughout hospitalisation and after discharge.

On discharge, basic information and advice will be given by the keyworker to both patient and family (Figures 11.1 and 11.2), to forewarn them of any problems, for example itching, insomnia, restlessness and swelling that may occur, and to give ideas that may help them to cope with and overcome those problems. There may also be days when the individual feels that he is functioning normally and others when he feels inadequate as provider, spouse or parent.

The individual will regularly attend the Burns Outpatient clinic in the first couple of weeks after discharge. It is important that, at these appointments, the keyworker, the outpatient nurse and patient are in contact with each other, so that adjustments to discharge can be discussed and emotions and inabilities expressed.

The experienced nurse will then be able to reassure the individual and recognise the need for other professionals, such as a psychiatrist or a child psychologist, to be involved if adjustments are becoming difficult (the individual's consent being needed first).

Behaviours that may indicate that the individual's mechanisms to cope are not being achieved are:

- Lack of compliance with burn aftercare
- Failure to attend scheduled appointments
- Unrealistic expectations concerning physical appearance and functional abilities

Once the patient has healed, it is important that he keeps in close contact with the keyworker, the outpatient nurse and the Burns Unit. Research shows that, even after being discharged for 2 years, an individual may still suffer psychosocial problems (Wallace, 1988).

Children's Discharge Advice Sheet

Sunshine

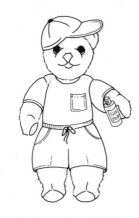

Your damaged skin is very sensitive.

Avoid sunshine
- Keep covered with cotton clothes
- Wear a hat
- Wear a total sunblock/high factor sun cream to burns, grafts and donor sites

Pressure Garments

It is important to wear your pressure garments for up to 2 years, to help flatten your scars.

Remove garments only to bathe/wash then massage in moisture cream to keep skin moist and supple before putting garments back on.

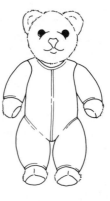

Swimming

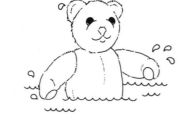

Swimming helps you to exercise your limbs when all your wounds are healed.

After swimming
- Shower to wash off all the chlorine
- Apply moisture cream
- Put pressure garments on

Fig 11.1   Children's discharge advice sheet

The current treatment of burns and scalds is aimed at the reduction of scarring, preventing disability, reducing the need for further surgery, and producing a better cosmetic result.

It is not necessary for all burn injuries to be treated by skin grafting. If your burn has healed without a skin graft, follow the care for a donor site when you go home.

Skin graft care

Unless the graft is fully healed when you leave hospital, you will be required to attend as an outpatient for further wound care. Once the wound is healed, normal personal hygiene should continue, and the skin graft site will require special care to minimise scarring and prevent it from becoming dry and itchy. In order to stop this occurring, the grafted area must be washed with non-perfumed soap (e.g. 'Simple' or baby soap) three times daily, then patted dry – do not rub the graft. After washing, moisturising lotion, again non-perfumed (e.g. aqueous cream) should be firmly massaged into the skin graft site in a circular movement to soften the scar tissue and to moisturise the graft site. It is necessary to continue this for at least 1 year, or longer if the skin graft becomes dry.

Donor site care (or care of a burn that has healed without a skin graft)

This is where the skin graft has been taken from – usually the thigh or the buttocks. It normally heals 7–10 days after the operation. Once it is healed and exposed, it should be washed and moisturised as for a skin graft (see above), or else it will become dry and itchy. The moisturising and massaging should continue until the area returns to normal skin colour.

Pressure garments

If you have had a skin graft, you may be required to wear an elastic garment to prevent hard, red, itchy scars, to flatten the graft and to improve the final appearance; this may depend on the area of the body skin grafted.

On discharge, you will be given a provisional garment, usually of Tubigrip, as permanent ones have to be ordered. When your wounds have healed, the occupational therapist will measure you for a pressure garment. This will need to be worn continuously for a period of 12–18 months to achieve the best possible results, and should only be removed for personal hygiene and laundering.

Pressure garments should be hand-washed in washing-up liquid or soap flakes – not soap powder (as this damages the elastic fibres) – and dried naturally away from heat (do not iron). Spare ones will be provided to allow for washing.

Sunshine

During the first 12 months after a burn injury, whether or not a skin graft has been required, the area of damaged skin will need to be protected from the sun, as it is very sensitive to the sun's rays and may blister even if exposed to mild sunshine.

Our advice is that all the areas of damaged skin should be covered when in sunlight for the first year. For areas that are naturally exposed, e.g. the face and hands, we recommend the use of total sunblock creams. The following year a 'high factor' sun cream is required for any exposed areas, and in the third year after injury, with care, you should be able to tolerate the sun as normal, applying a medium factor sun cream.

If you have any questions or problems when you have been discharged from hospital, do not hesitate to contact the Burns Unit. They are always willing to help, even if you just want someone to talk to. A self-help group is available to offer advice, and if you feel you would like to become a member to nelp others who have suffered burn injuries, please contact the Burns Unit directly.

Fig 11.2   Burns Unit discharge information for adults

STAGE 6: HOME VISITS

Those patients who were originally assessed as having major burns will also receive a home visit and, if applicable, a school visit from the keyworker and/or the out-patient nurse.

The home visit usually takes place around the eighth week after discharge. The purpose of this visit, as suggested by Manger and Speed (1986), is to:

- Evaluate the social reintegration of the burn patient
- Identify any problems that may need further assistance from the multi-disciplinary burns team
- Provide support for both patient and family
- Continue health promotion teaching

Activities of the patient are assessed, and relationships with other family members and friends are discussed. Referrals, if required, can be made through the Burns Unit.

The home visit provides an informal environment, which is more personal and relaxing for both patient and family. Problems are more likely to be expressed and solved before they become a major crisis in the rehabilitation of the patient.

If there are major problems, it may be necessary to repeat the home visit within the next couple of months, to ensure that coping mechanisms have been established.

STAGE 7: SCHOOL VISITS (PRE-SCHOOL ENTRY)

Once the child has been discharged from hospital, the main goal, as stated by Manger et al (1987), is 'to help the child transfer from the sheltered environment of the hospital back to the community'. This can only be achieved effectively by the child returning to school. The aim of the school visit is to:

- Prepare the school teachers, school nurse and children for the problems and anxieties that may occur for the burn-injured child and family in the rehabil-itation phase of care
- Provide practical information for both teachers and pupils, so that they can understand and cope with the burn-injured child
- Identify any problems, for example sports or cookery, that may affect the child on returning to school.

The keyworker and/or the outpatient nurse will visit the school either before the child returns to school or within the first week of attendance. After the initial meeting with the staff and school nurse, which outlines the reason for the visit, a leaflet on aftercare, physical, social and psychological care is given. Then a meeting with the children will take place. The actual content of this informal talk will vary depending on the developmental age of the children. Open discussion is encouraged, so that the children feel they can express any feelings or anxieties that they may have.

EVALUATION

The stages of the social reintegration programme are not set rigidly at fixed intervals. Individual plans of care, specific to the needs of the burn patient and family, are adapted to coincide with the physical programme of recovery.

The programme provides structure, accountability and support, which is needed for the patient's successful psychosocial recovery and reintegration into his previous environment.

Burn patients are individuals with differing problems, social reintegration is very dependant on social and cultural status. The Nottingham reintegration programme is the ideal and perhaps other Burns Units, with these guidelines may work towards the optimum social and cultural reintegration programmes their patients require.

BURNS UNIT SELF HELP GROUP

The Burns Unit also has a self help group B.U.S.H. This is a self help group formed by and available for patients, ex-patients, parents of children and also relatives. The group has been successful in arranging social events, fund-raising, support of newly burn injured patients and as a listening ear for parents, relatives and carers. No doubt there are problems which no amount of professional or self help support can change (Wallace, 1988). However, such services are provided to help individuals come to terms with the consequence of their injuries, and is part of the concept of psychological care.

References

Campbell L (1976) Special behavioural problems of the burned child. *American Journal of Nursing* **76**(1): 220–224.

Department of Health (1991) *Patient's Charter.* London: HMSO.

Douglas J (1993). *Psychology and Nursing Children.* London: Macmillan.

Manger G and Speed EA (1986) A coordinated approach to the discharge of burned children. *Journal of Burn Care and Rehabilitation* **6**(2): 127–129.

Marvin MT and Seligman R (1991) Psychosocial care of the burn patient and significant others. In: Trofino RB (ed.) *Nursing Care of the Burn Injured Patient*, pp 99–110. Philadelphia: FA Davis.

Mendelssohn I (1984) *Pain and Psychological Stress Management in Rehabilitation of the Burn Patient.* New York: Churchill Livingstone.

Partridge J (1991) *Changing Faces.* London: Penguin.

Wallace L (1988) Abandoned to a 'social death?' *Nursing Times* **84**(10): 34–37.

Manger G, Rahim N and Zettel Z (1987) Home and school visits by the burn unit nurse. *The Canadian Nurse* (Dec): 24–26.

12

Burns Aftercare and
Scar Management

This chapter explores aspects of rehabilitation that concern the treatment of burn scarring and its emotional effects on the patient's recovery. The term 'patient' is used throughout for convenience and continuity, but it is important to remember that one of the occupational therapist's most important roles is in facilitating the vital transition from patient to independent, functioning member of the community.

The development of unsightly scarring is a common sequela to the healing of burned skin, and one which can pose major problems to the patient in the long process of rehabilitation. Although one of the purposes of skin grafting is to minimise scarring, scars do develop in grafted areas, as they do in burns that have been treated conservatively but have taken more than 2–3 weeks to heal. Even donor sites may scar if the skin taken is anything other than extremely thin.

The scarring that occurs following burn injury is termed *hypertrophic*, which means literally 'overgrowth'. It is characterised by being lumpy, hard, red and extremely itchy. Less commonly, *keloid* scars may develop; these resemble particularly severe hypertrophic scars but are different in that they overgrow the margins of the original injury and can be particularly difficult to treat. A combination of both hypertrophic and keloid scars can occur concurrently in the same patient.

AETIOLOGY

The development of hypertrophic scarring is not yet fully understood, but several factors have been identified in its occurrence and may point to those patients at particular risk. These include:

1. *Age* – Children and adolescents tend to scar more severely than do adults.

2. *Site of burn* – Certain parts of the body are more prone to develop thickened scars, for example the chest and shoulders.

3. *Hair colour* – People with red hair seem to be particularly at risk.

4. *Race* – Fair skin and, conversely, very dark skin is predisposed to hypertrophic scarring.

5. *Infection* – The presence of infection delays healing and increases the chance of scar development (Lawrence, 1987).

6. *Type of graft* – Split-skin grafts scar more than do full thickness grafts.

7. *Genetic factors* – There appears to be a genetic link in scar development in many people, and a previous history of scarring may indicate a susceptibility.

PATHOLOGY OF SCAR FORMATION

Complex cellular activity in the healing skin can lead to a change from 'well-taken' graft to active, hypertrophic scar in a very short time. During healing, fibroblasts migrate into the wound and start to synthesise collagen. The normal process of collagen synthesis/lysis is interrupted, so that excessive collagen is deposited in lumpy whorls rather than the usual elongated fibres.

Some of the fibroblasts become modified to form myofibroblasts; these have the properties of smooth muscle cells and lead to a contraction of the scar tissue. During this stage, which can last for several months, the scar is termed 'immature'. It is initially quite fragile, but rapidly becomes raised, thickened and hard (Plate 11). The colour may vary from deep red to purple. Itching may be severe and prolonged. Scar contraction can be particularly aggressive and, if the scar extends across a joint, can lead to the development of deformity in a very short time. It can take up to 18 months, and occasionally longer, for the scar to become mature, at which time it will appear pale, contraction will have ceased and the itching will have subsided.

TREATMENT

At the present time, hypertrophic scarring cannot be prevented, but its effects can be minimised. Several treatment methods are available, and the therapist must make an early assessment of the healing wounds in order to plan the programme of treatment with the patient. Controlling the growth of scar tissue in its immature phase can produce a flatter, softer, more cosmetically acceptable scar. Controlling the contraction of scar tissue can prevent the development of disabling and unsightly deformities, and the need for corrective surgery.

Non-surgical methods of management available to the therapist include pressure therapy (Van Straten and Mahler, 1984), massage, the use of silicone gel sheets and elastomers, and splinting. These will be considered in some detail as they constitute the mainstay of treatment in Burns Units throughout the UK.

Pressure Therapy

The use of pressure in the treatment of deforming scars and contractures was documented as long ago as the late 17th century. Pressure has been used in a number of forms, including elastic bandages and adhesive plaster, with varying degrees of success throughout the centuries since then (Linares et al, 1993). Universal support for pressure therapy was only gained following the pioneering work of Duane Larson and his team (Larson et al, 1971) at the Shriners Burn Institute in America in the late 1960s. Further research by Kischer and others (Kischer et al, 1971; Haq and Haq, 1990) confirmed pressure therapy as a widely accepted first-line treatment for hypertrophic scarring.

Although its mode of action is not yet proved, it has been postulated that a regimen of continuous pressure of at least capillary level (25 mmHg) effects a realignment of the collagen bundles and, by producing a mild hypoxia of the cells, may control the overexuberant collagen synthesis (Figure 12.1). Leung and Ng (1980) also demonstrated a reduction in the discomfort of itching when pressure garments were worn.

Pressure can be achieved simply by using cotton elastic tubing, such as Tubigrip, or ready-made garments of the same material, but made-to-measure garments of a Lycra material are more commonly used and may afford more even pressure (Plate 12). As soon as the grafts have healed, detailed measurements are taken and a decision as to the required style of garment is made. There are several pressure garment manufacturers in the UK, each providing their own measuring charts and tapes and a wide variety of styles to suit all needs. Delivery times vary, but most patients can be fitted with their first garments within a week of ordering. Care must be taken when the initial garments are applied, as newly healed grafts

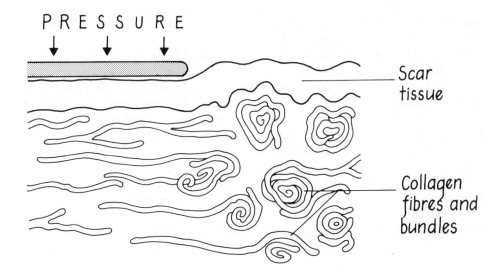

Fig 12.1   Hypertrophic scarring showing the effect of pressure

are fragile and must not be damaged in the process. Sometimes, a lower pressure is indicated for the first garments, and some manufacturers offer an 'interim' type of garment, which is used until the permanent ones are ready.

It is often best to order one set of garments only for the first fitting, as many patients request small changes, such as the positioning of zips, on the second garment. Patients should always return to the hospital when the first garments are ready; this ensures an accurate fit and provides an opportunity for the therapist to explain pressure therapy in more detail to the patient. Two sets of garments are normally provided, to allow for regular laundering. Although there are certain styles that are considered standard, the manufacturers offer an individual service so that not only are all garments made to measure, but particular deformities arising from contractures or amputations are also catered for. It is sometimes helpful for the therapist to include extra measurements, drawings and even photographs for an unusual request.

Some hospitals make their own pressure garments, usually for reasons of cost and convenience. Patients can be measured and fitted on the same day, which is particularly helpful if they live some distance from the hospital.

In order to be of maximum benefit, pressure therapy must be applied for an average of 23 hours per day, the garments only being removed for washing, bathing and creaming (Scott Ward, 1991). They are not always easy to wear, especially during hot weather, and patients need to keep in regular contact with their therapist to maintain motivation and compliance. Regular reassessments are also needed to determine the need for new garments and to re-measure as necessary, especially when the patient is a child.

Scarring of the face poses particular problems to both patient and therapist in the choice of an acceptable pressure technique. Semirigid, transparent, plastic facemasks fabricated from high-temperature thermoplastics are sometimes used. These can give excellent pressure, especially around the nose, where a fabric mask would not conform, but patients often find them hot to wear and uncomfortable for long periods (Rivers, 1979; Schons et al, 1981).

Inserts and conformers are sometimes used under garments to obtain pressure over 'difficult' areas. These include the palm of the hand, where the fabric bridges the anatomical arches, or around the nose, where the same occurs between the bony prominences of the cheek and the bridge of the nose. Conformers can be made simply from high density sponge, or for a more definitive mould, from a medical grade elastomer such as silastic foam, silastic elastomer or otoform. They are also useful worn under pressure gloves in the web spaces, to prevent web creep, a common problem with hand burns.

Pressure garments are discontinued when the scars are mature, normally 12–18 months post-burn. If no change in the scar is observed when the pressure garment is left off for 24 hours, the scar is deemed mature. If pressure therapy has been continuous, the scar should be pale, soft and reasonably flat at this stage. It is occasionally necessary to continue the treatment for longer periods, perhaps up to 3 years.

Massage

Sebaceous glands, which provide the sebum necessary for oiling normal skin, are destroyed in deep partial thickness and full thickness burns. Since split-skin grafts contain no sebaceous glands, the grafted skin is liable to be dry, inelastic and easy to damage. As soon as the graft is healed, patients must be shown how to cream the skin. The process needs to be repeated at least three times a day during the stage of active scarring, as well as after bathing. Any non-perfumed, water-based cream, such as E45, aqueous cream or Nivea, may be used. Some patients like to use vitamin E cream or the oil from vitamin E capsules, but these are expensive, and there is no research to suggest that they are any more efficacious than the cheaper creams. Aromatherapy massage is being used in several units to reduce burns scar itching.

Initially, creams should be applied gently to prevent damage to the newly healed graft, but deeper massage should be started as the skin becomes stronger. Regular, deep massage is an essential part of aftercare; performed properly, it will improve the quality of the skin, aid softening and flattening of the scar tissue, and help to prevent skin breakdown.

While regular showering or bathing is indicated thoroughly to cleanse grafted skin, the bathing process can be very drying, especially if the water is too hot, and the addition of a bath emollient, such as Bath E45, can help to prevent excessive drying.

Silicones

The use of topical silicone gel in the treatment of burn scars is a relatively recent development but one that is gaining in popularity as an adjunct or alternative to pressure therapy. Sheets of silicone gel (Plate 13), a chemically inert, transparent, flexible material, were originally used for burn scars in Australia, by Perkins and others in 1982, in conjuction with pressure garments. Later research by Quinn (1987) in the UK demonstrated a softening of hypertrophic scars with silicone gel but the mode of action was not identified. Further studies (Ahn et al, 1989; Ahn et al, 1991; Perkin et al, 1982) show that the gel is efficacious in the prevention and treatment of scars, and that the effect does not depend on pressure. This makes it useful as a treatment for small scars that do not warrant a pressure garment.

Silicone gel is applied directly to the healed skin and secured with an adhesive tape, such as Mefix, or with Tubigrip. Alternatively, it may be used on larger scars in conjunction with pressure garments, where, for practical reasons, its use may be limited to areas that are particularly lumpy.

Many patients report that it soothes the irritation in their scars. It is easy to use and relatively inexpensive, and there are few side-effects. Occasionally, patients are unable to use it because it exacerbates itching, but this is usually because it has been applied for too long or too soon, or because of poor hygiene. Careful explanation of its recommended use usually prevents problems. The skin should be fully healed before it is used, and a gradual increase in the wearing time during the first week is the rule.

The skin should be clean and dry, and excess cream should be removed before the gel is applied. It must be removed daily and the gel itself washed before reuse. The same piece is used repeatedly until it disintegrates. Recent expansion of the market in silicone gel has produced variations of the original 4 × 4 inch sheets, to include an adhesive gel and a thinner, non-sticky silicone, which resembles thin, flexible plastic, and which does not disintegrate with repeated use.

Splinting

The need to wear splints frequently continues beyond discharge from the Burns Unit, and splints are commonly worn in conjunction with pressure garments for many months, as scar tissue matures. In assessing the potential for hypertrophic scar development, the therapist must look out for restrictions of joint movement. Any burn that extends across a joint is liable to lead to a deformity, commonly a flexion deformity, but certain areas are particularly at risk. These include the neck, axillary folds, elbow, knee, first web space and little finger. The scar tissue contracts insidiously, and deformities that may not have been apparent, or even anticipated, can develop surprisingly quickly when the patient is at home. Contractures are most likely to occur in the first 3 months, and frequent out-patient appointments are recommended during this period in order to monitor the situation. Splinting is indicated at the earliest sign of contracture, as it is much easier to prevent a deformity than to correct an existing one. At this stage, most splints are worn only at night, and perhaps during periods of rest in the day. The exception to this is the conforming neck collar, which is commonly worn virtually continuously during the first 6 months, and removed only for washing, creaming and exercising. A range of low-temperature thermoplastic materials is available, the therapist's choice depending on a number of factors, including conformability and strength.

Splint wearing is always combined with a programme of exercise, and the occupational therapist will liaise closely with the physiotherapist in developing a treatment regimen that is tailored to individual patient's needs. Where there is an existing contracture, it is often best to make the splint immediately after physiotherapy, when the joint has been stretched to its maximum. Deep massage and the application of silicone gel over the contracture for 30 minutes prior to making the splint may also help to soften the skin and allow a few extra degrees of movement. At this stage, the contracture is only of the skin and underlying soft tissues, and should respond well to treatment. As improvement is gained, the splint is altered (serial splinting), in order to maintain progress, and should continue to be worn even when full range of movement is achieved, since immature scar tissue will quickly cause the joints to revert to the contracted position.

Sometimes, a contracture can only be corrected with surgery, but even this does not guarantee permanent improvement, and post-release splintage is vital if the same depressing cycle is to be avoided.

Splints are commonly worn over pressure garments, or may be lined with sili-cone gel to afford a sustained softening of contracted tissue. Strapping is of particular importance as the straps themselves form an integral part of the splint. Ineffective strapping of a little finger extension splint, for example, can render the splint useless. For this reason, it is vital that the patient is fully conversant with the splint regimen – how and when to put it on, how long to wear it, the need to check for skin damage, and, of course, what it is hoped will be achieved. Since the patient will have been bombarded with information in this rehabilitative phase, it is helpful if splint regimens are written down as a ready reminder. Written instructions should never be meant to replace frequent outpatient appointments, however, and the patient needs to be reassured that help is available at the end of a telephone.

Other Treatment Methods

Scars occasionally remain resistant to pressure therapy, and the plastic surgeon may prescribe additional treatments to resolve particularly stubborn scars. Keloids respond less well to any type of treatment and, if surgically excised, have the tendency to recur.

Additional treatments include:

1. *Steroids* – applied topically as creams or adhesive tape, or by intralesional injection.

2. *Surgical excision* – usually considered when the scar is mature, as early exci-sion of an immature scar tends only to interrupt its progress. For keloids, intralesional excision, leaving a margin of scar tissue, seems to offer a better prog-nosis than does total excision.

3. *Radiotherapy* – this is rarely given. It damages the fibroblasts and helps to prevent exuberant scar tissue forming again. It needs to be given as soon as possible after the scar has been treated surgically, as either an excision and closure, or as shaving and grafting of the scarred area. Pregnant females are excluded from this group, but children may rarely be considered if the problem is particularly severe, for example keloid scarring on the face. There is a tiny risk of skin tumours developing following radiotherapy, and this needs to be balanced against the actual scar problem. Close liaison with a radiotherapist is essential with this form of treatment.

COSMETIC CAMOUFLAGE

Residual scarring can be the source of a great deal of emotional trauma, and a complete recovery, in terms of socialising, forming relationships and a return to employment, may not be achieved. This is particularly, but not exclusively, likely if the scars are highly visible and not normally covered by clothing. In these instances, cosmetic camouflage can be of great benefit. Often, it is not started until pressure garments are abandoned, but patients should be made aware of it at an early stage, so that they know that treatment does not end when the garments are taken off.

Camouflage is not simply a form of make-up; the art of choosing and applying the cover creams is taught by specially trained experts (Leveridge, 1991). Since 1975, the British Red Cross Society has trained volunteers in this field, and they offer a service in many hospitals, while in other units, nurses, occupational therapists and physiotherapists have taken on the role.

When patients have been shown how to apply the creams, they are able to obtain continuing supplies on prescription or by private purchase from several recognised firms. The creams are waterproof, which allows the wearer the freedom of swimming and bathing without fear of the scar becoming visible.

Unfortunately, not all scars can be completely disguised, particularly if there is altered skin texture or if the scar is lumpy. In these instances, some improvement, rather than resolution, is usually possible, and further counselling may be needed if the patient remains unhappy with the final result. For some people, cosmetic camouflage is used as a temporary aid in rebuilding self-confidence, while for others it remains an essential and everyday part of their lives. Either way, it can produce remarkable results, not only visually, but also in terms of improved self-esteem.

PATIENT EDUCATION

Prior to discharge, the patient has a bewildering number of staff, of all disciplines, from whom to ask advice. This situation changes suddenly on discharge, and it is not uncommon for the patient to feel unsure about aftercare during this period.

There are several ways of minimising problems, the first of which is to ensure that the patient has been informed of possible hypertrophic scar development prior to discharge. It is common for staff to enthuse about 'excellent graft take' in the early days, but alarming and worrying for the patient when this rapidly translates into a lumpy, thickened scar. Careful explanation of the process, showing 'before' and 'after' pictures, and visits from other patients wearing pressure garments can be employed and the therapist must liaise closely with the nursing staff to ensure that information is given as and when the patient is ready to take it.

Printed sheets and booklets designed to answer common questions can be a useful reference to the patient at home, together with telephone numbers for easy contact if help is required between outpatient appointments.

Immediately after discharge, outpatient appointments will be frequent, perhaps daily, as the patient requires dressings, physiotherapy and occupational therapy. However, as the need for frequent attendances diminishes, new problems are still liable to arise, and there is a continuing need for information and support. After the first 3–4 months, apart from the plastic surgeon's outpatient clinic, it is often the pressure garment clinic that remains the patient's primary link with the burns team. For this reason, it is the occupational therapist's role to provide continuing education and support and to act as a liaison between other team members if late problems arise, for example with the unit outpatient dressings nurse for skin break-down, or in requesting an early clinic appointment if a particularly aggressive contracture develops.

Patients' concerns regarding their burn scars are numerous; some of the commonly encountered topics are discussed below.

Itching

Itching is one of the most common and most annoying problems in the early months, and patients should be reassured that it is normal and will resolve. It can be eased by the wearing of pressure garments and by regular massage. Medication can be prescribed if it is particularly severe.

Massage

Patients often ask how long regular creaming is required on both donor and grafted areas. The results of irregular creaming can often be seen in patients' dry and flaky scars, and patient education in this area is particularly important. Conversely, some patients are overenthusiastic in their use of creams and may need to be cautioned to use only the amount necessary to lubricate the skin, as excessive build-up of cream can macerate the skin and shorten the life of pressure garments.

Blistering

The formation of blisters is quite common in the first 3–4 months after healing and, while considered normal, can be a source of anxiety to patients. They need to be reassured that good hygiene and the wearing of correctly fitting pressure garments are indicated to prevent blister formation. The guidance for manage-ment of existing blisters is to cover with a light, non-stick dressing secured by the pressure garment, but if larger, open areas or infection develops, the advice of the GP or Burns Unit should be sought.

Exposure to Heat, Cold and Sunlight

The body's ability to react to extremes of temperature is commonly affected by a burn injury, and patients frequently report that their scars feel more uncom-fortable, itchy or even painful during very hot or cold spells. In cold conditions, the advice is to wear extra layers of loose, warm clothing, to take particular care with extremities, and to limit time spent out of doors, if at all possible. In hot weather, frequent tepid showers may be necessary in order to keep cool. Patients are often tempted to leave off their pressure garments when it is very hot and may need extra support to maintain motivation.

Sunlight brings its own problems, and it is important that patients understand that their active burn scars must never be exposed to sunshine without protection, as they will be much more sensitive to the effects of the sun. In effect, this means avoiding direct sun for at least 1 year after the burn and wearing extra protective clothing, for example a hat, if they must stay outside. Unfortunately, pressure garments alone do not protect against the sun as they are 60% porous, but the use of a total sunblock, applied frequently, under garments should offer adequate protection. Patients often ask about the wisdom of foreign holidays in the first year after a burn, and it has to be said that very hot climates are probably best avoided if the area of burned skin is extensive and difficult to keep covered.

Swimming

Swimming is an excellent form of exercise post-burn and may be resumed as soon as all areas of skin are healed. Pressure garments may be kept on or removed while swimming, but if kept on must be rinsed well afterwards to eliminate chlorine or salt. Swimming should always be followed by thorough, careful drying and creaming.

Sport

Contact sports are best avoided while scars are active, especially if they are in vulnerable areas, for example the shins. Gentler forms of leisure exercise, such as yoga or keep-fit, can be resumed when the skin is healed, and the stretching involved will be beneficial.

Skin Colour

Patients frequently worry about the colour of their burn scars and the fact that the colour deepens when pressure garments are not worn, during bathing and on the legs while standing for long periods. They need reassurance that this is quite normal and is due to changes in the blood's circulation. It can be limited by wearing the pressure garments and avoiding standing still for too long.

Loss of pigment (hypopigmentation) is a different problem and may be extensive, especially in areas of partial thickness burn that were not grafted, as the melanocytes may still have been destroyed. Return of pigmentation is difficult to predict, but this is a concern that should not be underestimated. With time, improvement usually occurs, and, if incomplete, cosmetic camouflage may be indicated.

Return to Work

Some patients are concerned about returning to work while their scars are still active, while others worry that they will lose their jobs if they are away for too long. For others, ongoing compensation claims complicate the situation and make planning for the future difficult. Each situation must be judged on its own merits, but the nature of some jobs, for example jobs that require a lot of standing or which involve working in extremes of temperature, will make them obviously unsuitable for those who have suffered major burns. Patients may benefit from a work assessment in the Occupational Therapy Department of a Rehabilitation Unit, or by being referred to the Disablement Employment Adviser if retraining is indicated. Staff should not underestimate the importance of an early return to employment, not only for financial reasons, but also for the part it plays in restoring self-esteem.

Sometimes, a return to work is interrupted by the need for further surgical treatment, but patients should be encouraged to discuss the timing of their surgery with the plastic surgeon so that work disruption is kept to a minimum.

Scar Resolution

Many patients ask what their scar will finally look like, a question that is difficult to answer in the early months. Some grafts settle so well that they eventually look like normal skin, although the evidence of meshing may still be apparent. Other areas, commonly those that took longer to heal or became infected, do not completely lose their lumpy appearance. They resolve to become pale or even white, but with a shiny texture that is obviously different from that of normal skin. Even with pressure therapy, some of the more aggressive scars do not flatten completely. It is important to warn patients that they are likely to be left with some scars, but the therapist must judge how much information to give at any one time.

EMOTIONAL PROBLEMS IN SCAR MANAGEMENT

Little has been mentioned so far regarding the patient's emotional response to the onslaught of treatment regimens that extend far beyond the day of discharge from the Burns Unit.

Jorgensen and Brophy (1975) have described three stages of psychological recovery from burns, and it is the third, recuperative, stage that mostly concerns scar management. If there is noticeable disfigurement or dysfunction, the patient may fear leaving the safety of the Burns Unit, where their condition is accepted and understood. They face the stares and questions of strangers, which may be dreaded, particularly if the injuries were self-inflicted or if the accident involved the death of another person.

The occupational therapist will be increasingly involved around the pre-discharge period, preparing the patient in practical ways, such as measuring for the first pressure garments, encouraging independence in activities of daily living and in discussion with the patient and family to emphasise the importance of regular follow-up. At this stage, the patient can be gently prepared for the possibility of scarring, and future treatments can be outlined.

Reluctance to leave the security of the Burns Unit is normal, but part of the patient's treatment prior to discharge will be to attend the Occupational Therapy Department, perhaps for a kitchen assessment, and this may signal the first time that anyone other than the burns team and the patient's relatives have seen the burn wound. It is the first stage in a long process described by Malick and Carr (1982) as 'progressive desensitisation' to the reactions of others to the patient's superficial deformity and disfigurement.

Once home, the patient is faced with the long process of rehabilitation, with its regime of exercise, splintage, creaming and pressure garments. It does not help that the burn scars begin to look worse in the first few months. Withdrawal and even depression can follow, and this, in turn, leads to apathy and loss of motivation. During this stage, the patient is likely to need a great deal of support, information and encouragement. Meeting with other patients in an informal support network can be as valuable as staff support. Grumbles about splints and pressure garments between fellow 'sufferers' can act as a safety valve against giving up altogether, as long as patients are carefully matched. Therapists should monitor closely the patient's levels of motivation and emotional status, offer counselling if this is within their expertise, or refer to another team member, such as the clinical psychologist. Appointments to check pressure garments may be used as informal counselling sessions, and gentle probing can sometimes reveal hidden difficulties, such as sexual problems, persistent feelings of guilt or revulsion, sleep difficulties and alienation from other family members.

Finally, the sheer length of time of burn rehabilitation, sometimes many years, is something that depresses many patients at the outset. It is as if their lives will never return to normal. With support, advice and encouragement from the burns team, that need not be the case, and the close rapport that often develops between patients and staff is of benefit to both. Successful rehabilitation is marked by a gradual reduction of dependency on the staff as the patient gains confidence in resuming pre-burn interests and activities.

References

Ahn ST, Monafo WW and Mustoe TA (1989) Topical silicone gel: a new treatment for hypertrophic scars. *Surgery* **106**(4): 781–787.

Ahn ST, Monafo WW and Mustoe TA (1991) Topical silicone gel for the prevention and treatment of hypertrophic scar. *Archives of Surgery* **126**(4): 499–504.

Haq MA and Haq A (1990) Pressure therapy in treatment of hypertrophic scar, burn contractures and keloid: the Kenyan experience. *East African Medical Journal* **11**: 785–793.

Jorgensen JA and Brophy JJ (1975) Psychiatric treatment modalities in burn patients. *Current Psychiatric Therapies* **15**: 85–92.

Kischer CW, Linares HA, Dobrkovsky M et al (1971) Electron microscopy of the hyper-
    trophic scar. In: *29th Annual Proceedings of the Electron Microscopy Society of America*,
    p 302. Boston: Claitor's Publishing Division.
Larson DL, Abston S, Evans EB et al (1971) Techniques for decreasing scar formation
    and contractures in the burned patient. *Journal of Trauma* **12:** 807–823.
Lawrence JC (1987) The aetiology of scars. *Burns* **13:** S3–S14.
Leung I and Ng M (1980) Pressure treatment for hypertrophic scars resulting from burns.
    Burns, Including Thermal Injury **6:** 244–250.
Leveridge A (1991) *Therapy for the Burn Patient*. London: Chapman & Hall.
Linares HA, Larson DL and Willis, Galstaun BA (1993) Historical notes on the use of
    pressure in the treatment of hypertrophic scars or keloids. *Burns Journal* **19:** 17–21.
Malick MH and Carr JA (1982) *Manual on Management of the Burn Patient*. Pittsburgh,
    PA: Harmaville Rehabilitation Center, Education Resource Division.
Perkins K, Davey RB and Wallis KA (1982) Silicone gel: a new treatment for burn scars
    and contractures. *Burns* **9:** 201–204.
Quinn KJ (1987) Silicone gel in scar treatment. *Burns* **13:** S33–S40.
Rivers E, Strate RG and Solem LD (1979) The transparent face mask. *American Journal
    of Occupational Therapy* **33:** 100–113.
Schons AR, Rivers E and Solem LD (1981) A rigid transparent face mask for control of
    scar hypertrophy. *Annals of Plastic Surgery* **6:** 245–248.
Scott Ward R (1991) Pressure therapy for the control of hypertrophic scar formation after
    burn injury. A history and review. *Journal of Burn Care and Rehabilitation* **12**(3):
    257–261.
van Straten O and Mahler D (1984) Pressure garments in the control of hypertrophic scar-
    ring and rehabilitation of the burn patient: an occupational therapy approach. *Journal
    of Medical Science* **20:** 320–322.

Further Reading

Rivers E (1984) Management of hypertrophic scarring. In: Fisher SA and Helm PA (eds)
    Comprehensive Rehabilitation of Burns, pp 177–217. Baltimore: Williams & Wilkins.
Rudolf R (1987) Widespread scars, hypertrophic scars, and keloids. *Clinics in Plastic Surgery*
    14: 253–260.

13

Psychological Care
following Burn Trauma

Burn injuries, a unique form of trauma, are in many respects the worst of all injuries that an individual can experience (Wachtel et al, 1983). In the UK, approximately 132 000 people per year receive hospital treatment for burns and scalds, and around 300 people die from their injuries (Home Office Statistics; Home Accident Surveillance System, 1987).

The increasing survival rate of burns victims is the result of major advances in the critical care of burns (Feller et al, 1979; Curreri et al, 1980). However, a consequence of this reduced mortality is an increase in a new type of morbidity: the physical and psychological problems experienced by burn survivors (Ward et al, 1987).

The first detailed account of the psychological consequences experienced by victims of severe burns were described following the Cocoanut Grove fire disaster in Boston, Massachusetts (Adler, 1943). Since then, a succession of studies has been undertaken following the same theme, which have been reviewed by Malt (1980) and Tucker (1986). A main unequivocal finding in all of these studies is that burn injuries precipitate serious psychological distress. The distress may be minimal or remedial if well-timed and structured psychological care is integrated as part of burn management during the course of hospitalisation.

Psychological care means that expressed or anticipated needs are responded to, rather than being ignored, belittled, attacked or judged (Cresci, 1982). The basic assumption of psychological care is the recognition and acceptance that all behaviour is determined by previous experience, by those factors of which the patient is aware, and by attitudes, conflicts and perceptions, of which the patient is totally unaware.

According to Cresci (1982), if consistent, appropriate psychological care on a Burns Unit is to be provided, then there are four basic requirements. First, all members of the multidisciplinary team should possess the ability to observe family, adult and staff reactions in an objective, non-judgmental manner. Second, part of the patient's admission process should include an assessment of the family system, for example marital relationships, decision-making, previous coping mechanisms and response to injury. This will enable predictions of the patient and family's adjustment to injury, surgery and hospitalisation. The third factor is the ability of the staff to empathise. Avoiding emotional contact or becoming overly protective will demonstrate a lack of understanding by staff of patients' needs. Fourth, a working knowledge of factors predisposing to a burn injury, the psychological reactions and adaptations, and the stages of recovery through which the patient and the family will evolve, must be acquired.

A combination of these four requirements seeks to provide members of the multidisciplinary team with a basic framework to guide the psychological care of patients following a burn injury during the course of hospitalisation and beyond.

Throughout the course of this chapter, the author will focus on individuals prone to a burn injury, psychological reactions and the stages of recovery in more detail, concluding with a section on the importance of effective communication in psychological care and possible strategies and solutions for the future.

FACTORS PREDISPOSING TO A BURN INJURY

Evidence in the literature suggests that some individuals are prone or predisposed to burn injuries (MacArthur and Moore, 1975).

A study undertaken by Noyes et al (1979) focused on the relationship between stressful life events and burn injuries. The results indicated that over a 1-year period, 50% of adults admitted to a Burns Unit had a pre-existing history of physical and/or psychiatric conditions that had increased their susceptibility to the burn injury. Many of the individuals were also found to be unemployed, single and from poor socio-economic circumstances, and reported a significant increase in stressful life events in the year preceding the injury.

Steiner and Clark (1977) indicated that post-burn psychiatric conditions developed more frequently among patients who had a previous psychiatric history, and Bowden et al (1980) pointed to a high incidence of burns among alcoholics. In 1983, Kolman also suggested that a large number of adults admitted to a Burns Unit came from disturbed family backgrounds, with unemployment, marital disharmony and poor housing conditions.

The results of these studies, therefore, suggest that, in many cases, burn injuries have their roots deep in the family setting, and imply that burn injuries may not always be purely accidental (Cresci, 1982). Individuals are often from dysfunctional depressed family settings, in which there may have been changes in the balance and structure of the family, such as a change in employment status, financial problems, a geographic move, divorce, remarriage, pregnancy or a physical or psychiatric illness prior to the burn injury.

Ward et al (1987) suggested that it is more often the person rather than the injury that determines the emotional prognosis after burn trauma. It is worth bearing this fact in mind when dealing with individuals who present with poor coping strategies, inadequate psychological adjustment or major psychological dysfunctions during the course of hospitalisation (Tobiasen and Hiebert, 1985; Buckhart, 1981; Roberts et al, 1987).

PSYCHOLOGICAL REACTIONS FOLLOWING A BURN INJURY

For those readers who may be unfamiliar with the psychological effects of burn injuries, this section seeks to outline the psychological reactions of an adult following a severe burn injury during the course of hospitalisation.

To be severely burned is both physically and emotionally a devastating experience (Noyes et al, 1971), and the individual concerned may experience extreme psychological reactions, which may compound the physical injury. It is an important part of psychological care that these reactions are understood and interpreted by members of the multidisciplinary team as part of the patient's normal defence and healing mechanisms (McGookin, 1991).

Because of the terrifying experience of the accident, the overwhelming events that follow, being rushed into hospital and the disorientation in an unfamiliar environment, it is not surprising that the patient is anxious and emotional on admission. However, it is worth noting that, at this stage, the patient may also be lucid, mentally clear and rational, even if he has sustained a major burn injury.

The physical appearance of the individual may be unpleasant, and members of the multidisciplinary team need to appreciate that relatives and other visitors who may come into contact with the patient will require considerable support and reassurance throughout.

The psychological reactions displayed by the patient are finite, temporary and often expected responses to the injury, and will resolve as the patient makes a physical recovery and becomes more independent. These reactions include withdrawal, denial, regression, anger or hostility, anxiety and depression.

Withdrawal is common in the acute phase of a burn injury, especially if it is severe or life-threatening, and the patient will show little interest in family, friends or external events.

Denial is a defence mechanism and may involve the individual denying the extent of the injury, loss of function, loss of life or injury to others. This protective defence mechanism relieves anxiety and external reality in the early stages (Blumenfield and Schoeps, 1993).

Regression is a normal adaptive mechanism, in which the individual may return to an earlier way of behaving or reacting in response to stress. According to Andreasen et al (1972b), the manifestations of regression are low tolerance to frustration, demanding, infantile behaviour, hypochondriasis, poor emotional control, obstructiveness and exaggerated dependency needs, and members of the multidisciplinary team may be angered by the display of manipulative behaviour. Unsympathetic management, hostile reactions or joining in the patient's games will, however, only reinforce the behaviour. On the other hand, being overly concerned may promote regression to child-like behaviour.

Anger and hostility may continue from the time of the injury to full recovery, the basis of the anger being loss or threatened loss, and this is part of the grief response. The patient may not be aware of angry feelings and repress them, turning them inward as depression, or he may project them or displace them onto another person.

Anxiety emerges because the individual experiences the injury as a dangerous situation that reawakens basic fears and threats encountered during early child-hood development (Blumenfield and Schoeps, 1993). Many of the feelings of anxiety come from the unconscious and relate to loss of body integrity, depen-dence, separation from family and friends, and loss of love and approval, or may be experienced as a punishment for previous transgressions (Blumenfield and Schoeps, 1993).

Depression is an expected response to any loss or threatened loss. Patients may verbalise sadness, are tearful, and show a poor appetite, weight loss, sleep distur-bances and decreased self-esteem.

Differing personality styles can also be related to individuals' reactions to injury. Kahana and Bilbring (1968) described seven basic personality types in terms of psychological reactions: oral, compulsive, hysterical, masochistic, paranoid, schizoid and narcissistic. Recognising individuals with a predominantly fixed style will allow members of the multidisciplinary team to understand patient/staff inter-actions that may occur during the stages of recovery.

In adults, the feelings of frustration, resentment and guilt experienced during the period of hospitalisation may produce an unco-operative and obstructive patient, leading to violent outbursts, abuse of staff and refusal of treatment. Responding with kindness and sympathy, combined with firmness, should be rewarded by successful management (Cason, 1981).

ADAPTATION AND STAGES OF RECOVERY

Watkins et al (1988) developed a seven-stage method of assessing and assisting burn victims' psychological recovery. Each stage consisted of a dynamic reaction between cognitive (thinking) and affective (feeling) processes, resulting in the indi-vidual displaying adaptive behaviour, along with the most appropriate staff intervention.

Adaptive stages include: survival, anxiety, pain, a search for meaning, recuper-ation, acceptance of loss, rehabilitation and reintegration of identity. Staff interventions include: orientation, medication, validation, education, legitimisation, commendation and termination.

Cresci (1982) and Price (1990) describe the course of recovery in three phases: shock stage, immediate stage and rehabilitation.

The shock stage/acute phase coincides with the first 48–72 hours post-injury, when the patient is acutely ill and receiving treatment designed to support body organ function and fluid and electrolyte balance. At this stage, the patient is often disorientated or may be unconscious (Price, 1990). The effects of the burn injury, and the sensory and sleep deprivation associated with ongoing treatments, serve to prevent the patient from orientating himself to the environment (Paterson, 1987).

The individual may appear anxious, confused, frightened and frustrated, experiencing periods of agitation, hostility, denial and disorientation to time and place. Treating the underlying causes should alleviate these reactions (Cresci, 1982). Members of the multidisciplinary team should aim to provide simple information and orientation to the environment and treatment carried out, while anticipating hidden fears.

Relatives may also present acute grief reactions and guilt. Involvement in care will help to reduce helplessness, and encouraging ventilation of feelings and emotions will assist with communication and building up a therapeutic relationship.

The intermediate stage/healing phase comprises the following 2–6 weeks and coincides with intensive wound care management and the start of rehabilitation. At this stage, the patient focuses on pain and discomfort (Price, 1990) and, as time progresses, becomes more aware of the extent of the burn injury. Emotional outbursts, despair, hopelessness, grief and mourning over losses are evident. Relatives may feel unable to deal with these outbursts and are unsure how to respond. Members of the multidisciplinary team should seek to encourage and support relatives and friends in providing active involvement, reassurance and support.

The rehabilitation stage, which begins with the end of the initial surgical procedures and extends to discharge from hospital and future care is the third stage. At this point, the patient re-establishes physical and psychological independence. In the short term, the individual may feel isolated or unloved, as people react to the injuries with fear, alarm or withdrawal. Discharge plans are formulated in accordance with individual patient needs and also those of the family or carers. Whenever possible, social reintegration programmes should be arranged prior to discharge, to allow the opportunity and experience of meeting people outside the Burns Unit and be observed by others, to develop new skills in accepting a change in body image, and to enhance socialisation skills for the future.

Noyes et al (1971) commented that 'patients who have been exposed to the experience of a severe burn injury and recover without serious psychological sequelae is moving testimony to the strength of the human adaptive potential'.

Understanding psychological processes in burn victims is still a relatively unexplored aspect of burn care and rehabilitation (Watkins et al, 1988). Reaction, adaptation and recovery should be viewed as a continuous process throughout the course of hospitalisation and discharge and, in some cases, for several years after the burn injury.

EFFECTIVE COMMUNICATION IN PSYCHOLOGICAL CARE

This final section focuses on the importance of effective communication in the psychological care of individuals following a burn injury. It seeks to identify the problems encountered by nursing staff on one Burns Unit, analyses them, and suggests possible strategies and solutions that could be realistically implemented in clinical practice to improve the quality of psychological care for the future.

The psychological aspects of burn patients' care are far-reaching (McGookin,

1991). The burns nurse requires a sound foundation in these matters, together with a variety of effective interpersonal and counselling skills, thus complementing the Burns Unit's multidisciplinary efforts to minimise psychological distress and facilitate the healing process. Therefore, communication is crucial for effective psychological care, because effective communication is the key to its achievement (Hyland and Donaldson, 1989).

A move towards primary nursing in the Nottingham Burns Unit made nursing staff more aware of their roles and responsibilities in providing holistic care on an individual basis. Great emphasis was placed on maintaining high standards of physical care, but the psychological needs of patients were not met, for a variety of reasons: scant attention was paid by nurses when attempting to assess psychological vulnerability in patients early in the course of hospitalisation; a nursing model and documentation that emphasised physical rather than psychological care were used; there were constraints within the clinical setting in terms of time and priorities of care; perceived levels of good interpersonal skills were low; there was a lack of previous or adequate training in using therapeutic interventions; and patient interactions were identified as brief, ad hoc and superficial. On the basis of the problems identified, the situation was analysed.

Evidence in the literature suggests that some individuals are more prone or predisposed to burn injuries (Mac Arthur and Moore, 1975). However, a review of the literature indicated the paucity of any appropriate assessment tools or strategies that could be used by nurses in the Burns Unit in order to highlight individuals at risk of psychological distress early in the course of hospitalisation.

A review of adult admissions to the Burns Unit positively illustrated a variety of factors. Some patients, more specifically than others, appeared to have contributed to the occurrence of the burn injury, and not all the injuries appeared to be accidental. In several, a significant emotional crisis or major change in the pattern of living preceded the injury.

The nursing model and documentation in use was that of Roper et al (1980), which is directed towards physical rather than psychological care. This appeared only to encourage a superficial level of questioning. There were no structured patient assessments, and little opportunity was given to allow patients to divulge either social or psychological concerns. The nature of the documentation also did not allow for the provision of written evidence of any nurse–patient interactions relating to psychological care that had taken place, and of the resulting outcomes.

The clinical setting was the next target. Sathe (1983) suggests that the organisational culture might not encourage nurses to invite patients to talk about their problems or promote what Cassee (1975) called an open, two-way communication.

Reflecting on the clinical situation and the realities of managing the severely burned patient amid the typical pressures present in a busy specialist unit, the problems of lack of time, heavy workloads and perceived priority constraints were seen to influence the degree to which nurses were prepared to be facilitative in their interventions towards patients. A small number of nurses felt that psychological care was of paramount importance and that, in the long run, time thus invested was time well spent. That view was neither universally held nor understood by others, and, in some cases, nurses felt that psychological care should be secondary to the more pressing needs of physical care.

In an attempt to assess the interpersonal skills of nurses within the unit, self-perceptions of interpersonal skills were recorded. Using Heron's (1986) six category intervention analysis, nurses were asked to rank order six intervention categories in terms of their perceived level of skills. The six categories are prescriptive (offering advice or making suggestions), informative (giving information or instruction), confronting (challenging the person's behaviour, attitudes or beliefs), cathartic (enabling the release of tension and strong emotions), catalytic (drawing out and encouraging further self-exploration) and supportive (validating or confirming the other person's self-worth).

The majority of nurses described themselves as being more skilled in informative, supportive and prescriptive roles and least skilled in being catalytic, cathartic and confronting.

In general, these results reflected those of similar studies undertaken by Burnard and Morrison (1988) and Morrison and Burnard (1989), and supported Heron's (1975) statement that a wide range of practitioners in our society show a greater deficit in the skilful use of facilitative interventions (cathartic and catalytic) than they do in the skilful use of authoritative namely prescriptive and informative, ones. According to Morrison and Burnard (1993), the reason for this may be that the facilitative approach takes time.

Catalytic, cathartic and confronting approaches involve an assessment of self that may be emotionally draining. The majority of nurses had also not received training, either pre- or post-registration, in therapeutic interventions or in how to cope with the expression of personal problems and emotion. This view was reflected in studies undertaken by the Joint Board of Clinical Nursing Studies (1981), now the English National Board of Post Basic Studies, which found that, in most courses, communication was not taught in any structured way. However, interpersonal skills training continues to be an important aspect of nurse education today (Kagan, 1985; MacLeod Clark and Faulkner, 1987; Burnard, 1989).

In physically observing staff in their interactions with patients, it was possible to determine a lack of skills in maintaining effective interaction, for example in using closed and leading questions, distancing themselves from patients, performing brief and superficial interactions, and blocking potentially difficult information as they appeared unsure how to deal with it, thereby preventing patients sharing concerns and absently ignoring patient cues. A general fear among nurses appeared to be that if they encouraged patients to disclose problems, strong emotions that they would be unable to deal with might be provoked. If effective communication is the tool of psychological care (Hyland and Donaldson, 1989), communication in the psychological care of individuals following burn trauma would be more effective by implementing the following strategies and solutions.

Owing to the paucity of any assessment tools, the first aim was to design an assessment tool in the form of a semi-structured questionnaire that could be used by nurses in the unit as part of burn care management, as a measure to assess and predict patients who might be prone to psychological vulnerability (Bosworth and Regel, 1993). Factors influencing the design were gleaned by a review of the literature, especially an article by Andreasen et al (1972a), which sought to examine the relationship of pre-morbid emotional and physical factors to the adjustment of burn patients following injury and hospitalisation. The literature suggests that those patients who have adjusted poorly tended to have a greater frequency of changes or stresses in their life situation prior to the injury and implied that recent experience of major illness, accident or injury during life may be a contributing factor to adjustment during hospitalisation. This information was not routinely gained from patients nor previously seen as being significant.

The questionnaire is wide ranging and open ended, in order that, during its use, nurses may follow a question up with probes or prompts to encourage patients to go into more depth with their answers.

Given the sensitivity of the information, reliability is of utmost importance. Patients often give answers that they think the nurses want to hear, or do not disclose information they feel may put them in an unfavourable light. Consideration was also given to whether other measures or assessment tools of a general nature, for example the Beck Depression Inventory (Beck et al, 1979) or the Hospital Anxiety and Depression Scale (Zigmond and Snaith, 1983) might be used in conjunction.

The second aim was to use the assessment tool as part of an assessment process for each adult patient, to elicit specific information that was not routinely gleaned from the previous documentation. This could highlight pre-existing physical or psychiatric conditions that might have increased the patient's susceptibility to the injury, making them more prone to complications that might affect the eventual outcome (Noyes et al, 1979). It may also be used to aid predictions of how the patient and the family will adjust to injury, hospitalisation and surgery. Another possible solution was to consider an alternative to the Roper nursing model that would focus on psychological care, for example that of Roy (1984).

Within the time constraints on the unit, and using the questionnaire as part of an assessment process, another solution would be to plan a series of structured interviews on each adult patient, undertaken by the patient's primary or associate nurse and lasting for approximately 30 minutes, once or (as the patient's condition dictates) twice a week from admission to discharge. Individualised care, and in particular primary nursing, leads to a better relationship between the nurse and patient, as the patient is able to get to know and trust one nurse, who is therefore in a better position to provide psychological care (Hyland and Donaldson, 1989).

Providing psychological care means focusing on patients as people. Some nurses have a natural ability – they automatically listen, observe, empathise and communicate well – but most health-care professionals need to develop these skills (Faulkner, 1992). In order to undertake the patient interviews, a series of training sessions would be required to outline the process and train staff in the appropriate skills required.

Preparation for the patient interviews is important, as ensuring privacy and maintaining a safe environment assists patients in disclosing problems and concerns, which would not otherwise be possible (Faulkner, 1992). Nursing staff need to be assertive about their need for time and privacy with the patient and avoid interruptions that may break the flow of the interview. The structure of the Burns Unit allows the provision of single rooms, where confidential interviews may be carried out. The staff, through training, need to develop the verbal skills required for an effective interview as research suggests that most nurses do not exhibit the required skills (Faulkner, 1980; Macleod Clark, 1982). What is encouraging is that, in experimental studies, nurses improved their skills dramatically after brief training (Maguire, 1982; Faulkner and Maguire, 1984).

These relevant skills include employing an appropriate questioning style, for example open, closed or leading. An open question is one that does not restrict the respondent in any way and also allows expression of feelings. Closed questions give the patient a forced choice of answer but may be useful when facts are required. Leading questions are those which imply the preferred answer and, as such, are inappropriate in effective interactions (Faulkner, 1992). Other skills include encouraging precision and clarification, picking up cues, and at all times using a negotiating style that facilitates disclosure of current concerns. The nurse also needs to learn appropriate skilled opening and closing strategies, while maintaining effective control throughout the interview.

In the same way that verbal skills need to be developed to improve interaction between the nurse and patient, the importance of non-verbal interaction has been well documented (Argyle, 1988). These skills include listening, the active use of silence, touch, the significance of gestures, eye contact and posture.

If the patient's problems are to be identified in a skilled way during an interview, the encounter must be given structure and focus, together with a willingness on the part of the nurse to explore the patient's feelings, sometimes at a deep level, and to examine these without doing the patient any harm. On the part of the nurse, the need to negotiate, to assign some priority to the patient's cues and to control diversions, such that the focus is maintained until each sequence is closed, is required (Faulkner, 1992).

Helping patients to explore their feelings may help them to come to terms with these but, in doing so, a number of emotions may be elicited that would normally be suppressed or contained. Nurses may require further training on the appropriate interventions. Talking does not solve problems, but interactions can be therapeutic.

It is intended that the interviews will highlight areas of psychological vulnerability and coping responses, and will promote acceptance of injuries, improved understanding and more active involvement by the patient in treatment, pain relief and realistic preparation for the difficulties that may be encountered after discharge from hospital. Many emotional responses including anger, guilt, denial, fear, anxiety and sometimes depression and suicidal thoughts, will be encountered during the interviews. The nurse needs to build up a good therapeutic relationship with the patient in order to allow him to ventilate his feelings and to offer interventions.

Once the interview is complete, the information elicited should be recorded by the patient's primary or associate nurse on the appropriate documentation and stored in the patient's case notes, thereafter being reviewed by the supervising clinician at regular intervals and being up-dated after each interview.

Finally, in order to improve the low perceived levels of interpersonal skills high-lighted in the early stages of treatment, a further training programme, together with active supervision and support for staff, could be set up. It is envisaged that training would include the following theoretical and practical elements: basic infor-mation gathering, counselling skills, establishing a therapeutic relationship, relationship enhancement methods and role play (and related experiential tech-niques). Because of the potential problem of developing facilitative skills, some nurses may find that they become overinvolved in patients' problems, taking them home or feeling under stress because they, personally, cannot help. The provision of ongoing supervision and support is therefore essential.

The Unit has an identified psychiatrist, psychologist and psychotherapist, so one could be co-opted to the role of supervisor. Supervision is an important part of the learning process for anyone involved in counselling. Effective supervision provides support, monitoring of standards and personal opportunity to develop skills. People who work with other people's problems need care and support them-selves. Supervision provides that support and helps to develop a more professional role, which increases the potential of using knowledge in practice. These ideas are reflected in the studies by Worthington and Roehike (1971), Urbano (1984) and Dryden and Thorne (1991).

Until recently it was standard practice on the Burns Unit that regular staff support groups were held, facilitated by a psychotherapist. The purpose of these is to provide a forum for raising controversial issues and to help staff express and clarify their feelings with attitudes towards work, each other, themselves, the patients and the patients' families. They were also used to help staff develop new skills in communication. We expect to resume these sessions in the near future.

CONCLUSION

The growing recognition of the importance of the burn patient's psychological needs means that nurses must acquire a greater understanding of the processes involved in communicating with patients. Such an understanding may, in turn, facilitate an improvement in communication and provide holistic patient care.

Providing psychological care is an art, and the art of psychological care may be developed through experience (Hyland and Donaldson, 1989). If nurses empha-sise psychological care in their nursing approach to burn care, they will develop their own psychological skills, skills that can be used in other situations and which involve the ability to understand people, to form warm caring relationships, and to help others to achieve their goals.

Anyone who treats burn injuries has a professional and moral responsibility to investigate their cause. It is clear that there are no easy solutions to adjustment to a burn injury, but the patient's courage and confidence in his own abilities, and a well-planned, comprehensive approach by staff using effective communication skills to meet the patient's psychological needs, can soften the impact of the injury and assist in developing trust and security between the patient, his relatives and staff on the Burns Unit.

References

Adler A (1943) Neuropsychiatric complications in victims of the Boston Cocoanut Grove disaster. *Journal of the American Medical Association* **123**(17): 1098–1101.

Andreasen NJC, Noyes R and Hartford CE (1972a) Factors influencing adjustment of burns victims during hospitalisation. *American Journal of Psychosomatic Medicine* **34**(6): 517–520.

Andreasen NJC, Noyes R and Hartford CE (1972b). Management of emotional reactions in seriously burned adults. *New England Journal of Medicine* **286:** 65–69.

Argyle M (1988) *Bodily Communication*, 2nd edn. London: Methuen.

Beck AT, Rush AJ, Shaw BF and Emery G (1979) *Cognitive Therapy of Depression. A Treatment Manual*. New York: Guildford Press.

Blumenfield M and Schoeps MM (1993) Psychological reactions to burn and trauma. In: Blumenfield M and Schoeps MM, *Psychological Care of the Burn and Trauma Patient*, pp 94–121. Boston: Williams & Wilkins.

Bosworth C and Regel S (1993) The Psychological and Psychiatric Morbidity Questionnaire (PPMQ). A measure to assess and predict psychological and psychiatric morbidity in individuals following burn trauma. *Journal of Clinical Nursing* **2:** 373–379.

Bowden ML, Feller I, Tholen D et al (1980) Self esteem of severely burned patients. *Archives of Physical Medicine and Rehabilitation* **61:** 449–452.

Buckhart CS (1987) Coping strategies of the chronically ill. *Journal of Nursing Clinics of North America* **22:** 543–550.

Burnard P (1989) *Teaching Inter-personal Skills. A Handbook of Experiential Learning for Health Professionals*. London: Chapman & Hall.

Burnard P and Morrison P (1988) Nurses' perceptions of their interpersonal skills. A descriptive study using six category intervention analysis. *Nurse Education Today* **8:** 266–272.

Cason JS (1981) Psychological and psychiatric problems. In: Cason JS, *Treatment of Burns*, pp 266–272. London: Chapman & Hall.

Cassee ET (1975) Cited in: Cox C and Mead A (eds) *A Sociology of Medical Practice, Therapeutic Behaviour, Hospital Culture and Communication*, London: Collier Macmillan.

Cresci JV (1982) Emotional care of the hospitalised thermally injured. Cited in: Hummel R (1982) *Clinical Burn Therapy*, pp 475–507. Bristol: John Wright.

Curreri PW, Braun DW and Shires GT (1980) Burn injury: analysis of survival and hospitalisation time for 937 patients. *Annals of Surgery* **192:** 472.

Dryden W and Thorne B (1991) *Training and Supervision for Counselling in Action*. London: Sage.

Faulkner A (1980) The student nurse's role in giving information to patients. Unpublished MLitt thesis, University of Aberdeen. Cited in: Faulkner A (1992) *Effective Interaction with Patients*, pp 1–8. London: Churchill Livingstone: Edinburgh.

Faulkner A (1992) *Effective Interaction with Patients*, pp 27–37. Edinburgh: Churchill Livingstone.

Faulkner A and Maguire P (1984) Teaching assessment skills. Cited in: Faulkner A (ed.) (1984) *Recent Advances in Nursing Communication*, pp 61–67. Edinburgh: Churchill Livingstone.

Feller I, Crane K and Flanders S (1979). Baseline data on the mortality of burn patients. *Quality Review Bulletin* **7**(4): 4.

Heron J (1975) *Six Category Intervention Analysis*. Human Potential Research Project. Guildford: University of Surrey.

Heron J (1986) *Six Category Intervention Analysis*, 2nd edn. Human Potential Research Project. Guildford: University of Surrey.

Home Accident Surveillance System (1987) London: Department of Trade and Industry.

Hyland ME and Donaldson ML (1989) *Psychological Care in Nursing Practice*, p 2, 1976. London: Scutari Press.

Joint Board of Clinical Nursing Studies (1987) *General Nursing Council for England and Wales: A Report.* London: General Nursing Council.

Kagan C (1985) *Inter-personal Skills in Nursing Research and Applications.* London: Croom Helm.

Kahana RJ and Bilbring GL (1968) *Lectures in Medical Psychology*, p 246. New York: International Universities Press.

Kolman P (1983) The incidence of psychopathology in burned adult patients – a critical review. *Journal of Burn Care and Rehabilitation* **416**: 430–436.

Mac Arthur J and Moore F (1975) Epidemiology of burns. The burn prone patient. *Journal of the American Medical Association* **231**: 259–263.

McGookin C (1991) Psychological problems of the burned adult. Cited in: Leveridge A (1991) *Therapy for the Burn Patient*, pp 69–85. London: Chapman & Hall.

Macleod Clark J (1982) Nurse patient verbal interaction. Unpublished PhD thesis, University of London. Cited in: Faulkner A (1992) *Effective Interaction with Patients*, pp. 1–8. London: Churchill Livingstone.

Macleod Clark J and Faulkner A (1987) Cited in: Davis B (ed.) (1987) *Teaching in Nurse Education*. Nurse Education Research and Developments Communication Skills. London: Croom Helm.

Maguire P (1982) *Doctor Patient Skills in Social Skills and Health*. London: Methuen.

Malt U (1980) Long term psychological follow-up studies by burned adults. A review of the literature. *The Burns Journal* **6**: 190–197.

Morrison P and Burnard P (1989) Students and trained nurses' perceptions of their own interpersonal skills: a report and comparison. *Journal of Advanced Nursing* **14**: 321–329.

Morrison P and Burnard P (1993) *Caring and Communicating*, 3rd edn. London: Macmillan.

Noyes R, Andreasen NJC and Hartford CE (1971) The psychological reaction to severe burns. *American Journal of Psychosomatic Medicine* **11**: 416–422.

Noyes R, Frye SJ, Slymen DI and Canter A (1979) Stressful life events and burn injuries. *Journal of Trauma* **19**(3): 141–144.

Paterson R (1987) Psychological management of the burn patient. *Topics in Acute Care and Trauma Rehabilitation* **1**(3): 25–39.

Price B (1990) The burn patient. In: Price B, *Body Image Concepts and Care*, pp 183, 199. Hertfordshire: Prentice Hall.

Roberts JG, Browne G, Steiner D et al (1987) Analysis of coping responses and adjustment. Stability of conclusions. *Nursing Research* **36**(2): 94–97.

Roper N, Logan W and Tierney AJ (1980) Nursing and the activities of living. In: *The Elements of Nursing*, pp 73–280. Edinburgh: Churchill Livingstone.

Roy C (1984) Introduction to nursing – an adaptation model. Cited in: Aggleton P and Chambers H (1992) *Nursing Models and the Nursing Process*, pp 83–99. London: Macmillan.

Sathe V (1983) Implications of corporate culture – a manager's guide to action. *Organisational Dynamics* **12**: 5–23.

Steiner H and Clark WR (1977) Psychiatric complications of burned adults – a classification. *Journal of Trauma* **17**: 134–143.

Tobiasen JM and Hiebert JM (1985). Burns and adjustment to injury. Do psychological coping strategies help? *Journal of Trauma* **25**: 1151–1155.

Tucker P (1986) The burn victim – a review of psychosocial issues. *Australian and New Zealand Journal of Psychiatry* **20**: 413–420.

Urbano JM (1984) Supervision of counsellors. Ingredients for effectiveness. *Counselling* **50**: 7–16.

Wachtel TL, Kahn V and Frank HA (1983) Rehabilitation of the burn injured patient. *Current Topics in Burn Care*, pp 217–220. Rockville, MD: Aspen Systems Corporation.

Ward HW, Moss RL, Darko DF et al (1987) Prevalence of post burn depression following burn injury. *Journal of Burn Care and Rehabilitation* **8**(4): 294–297.

Watkins PN, Cook EL, May SR and Ehleben CM (1988) Psychological stages in adaptation following a burn injury. A method for facilitating psychological recovery of burn victims. *Journal of Burn Care and Rehabilitation* **9**(4): 376–384.

Worthington EL and Roehike HJ (1971) Effective supervision as perceived by beginning counsellors in training. *Journal of Counselling Psychology* **26**: 64–73.

Zigmond AS and Snaith RP (1983) The hospital anxiety and depression scale. *Acta Psychiatrica Scandinavica* **67**: 361–370.

14

Burn Trauma and

Post-traumatic Stress Disorder

'I did within these six days see smoke still remaining of the late fire in the City; and it is strange to think how this very day I cannot sleep at night without great terrors of fire, and this very night could not sleep until almost 2 in the morning through thoughts of fire.'

So recorded Samuel Pepys in his diary on the 18 February 1667, 6 months after the Great Fire of London in 1666 (Latham and Matthews, 1970–83). Pepys' account is perhaps one of the earliest thoroughly documented descriptions of a major disaster and its aftermath. His accounts of the fire and its psychological sequelae provide a detailed and fascinating account of his own, and others' reactions to the effects of the fire. There is also ample evidence to suggest from his accounts that he experienced symptoms of post-traumatic stress disorder (PTSD) (Daly, 1983).

Despite this, and many other earlier accounts (Trimble, 1985), the concept of PTSD was not officially recognised as a serious mental health problem until 1980, when it was included in the psychiatric diagnostic handbooks (American Psychiatric Association, 1980).

The American Psychiatric Association's 4th edition of its *Diagnostic and Statistical Manual of Mental Disorders* (DSM–IV) (American Psychiatric Association, 1994) has since been published, and in this edition, in order to meet the diagnostic criteria for PTSD, the requirements are that:

The development of characteristic symptoms following exposure to an extreme traumatic stressor involving direct personal experience of an event that involves actual or threatened death or physical injury, or other threat to one's physical integrity; or witnessing an event that involves death, injury or a threat to the physical integrity of another person; or learning about unexpected or violent death, serious harm, or threat of death or injury experienced by a family member or other close associate.

Furthermore, three distinct groups of symptoms are known to arise after a traumatic event: re-experiencing intrusive imagery, avoidant and arousal symptoms (Figure 14.1). In order to fulfil the complete diagnostic criteria for PTSD, the individual must experience at least one (or more) symptom from A, at least three (or more) from B and at least two (or more) from C. Previously, in order to meet the diagnostic criteria the individual must have 'experienced an event that is

A. **Re-experiencing symptoms**

1. Recurrent, intrusive, distressing recollections of the event, e.g., images, thoughts, or perceptions
2. Recurrent distressing dreams of the event
3. Acting or feeling as if the traumatic event were recurring (flashbacks)
4. Intense psychological distress at exposure to internal or external cues
5. Reactive physiological arousal to internal or external cues that symbolise or resemble an aspect of the trauma

B. **Circumscribed avoidance and dissociative mechanisms**

1. Avoidance of thoughts, feelings or conversations associated with the trauma
2. Avoidance of activities and situations
3. Inability to recall an important aspect of the trauma
4. Diminished interest and participation in significant activities
5. Feelings of detachment and estrangement from others
6. Restricted range of affect (e.g. unable to have loving feelings)
7. Sense of foreshortened future

C. **Heightened arousal**

1. Sleep disturbance
2. Irritability and anger
3. Concentration difficulties
4. Hypervigilance
5. Exaggerated startle response

Fig 14.1   Symptoms of PTSD

outside the range of usual human experience and that would be markedly distressing to almost anyone' (DSM–IIIR) (American Psychiatric Association, 1987). The exclusion of this is significant, as the implications for those suffering from burn trauma are twofold:

1.   The size or extent of the injury will not necessarily be an indication of whether the individual will develop symptoms of PTSD.

2.   There is an indication that the development of PTSD is often related to the way an individual interprets and makes sense of his experience, rather than to the experience per se.

THE EPIDEMIOLOGICAL EVIDENCE – A BRIEF REVIEW

While there are numerous references in the psychiatric and psychological literature to what we now know to be PTSD, it was research in the USA with Vietnam

War veterans which highlighted the syndrome and supplied much of the data on which the DSM–IIIR criteria were based (Blanchard et al, 1982). Since then, there has been considerable research into PTSD with rape victims (Burgess and Holmstrom, 1974; Foa et al, 1992; Rothbaum et al, 1992) and victims of disaster, most notably in the UK with the Bradford City Football Club fire (Duckworth and Charlesworth, 1988), the sinking of the *Herald of Free Enterprise* (Hodgkinson, 1990) and the King's Cross underground station fire (Sturgeon et al, 1991). In the USA, one of the worst fire disasters occurred in 1942 at Boston's Cocoanut Grove night-club, where a celebration turned to tragedy when a reveller accidentally set fire to an artificial palm tree. The fire, which spread suddenly, resulted in the deaths of almost 500 people. This disaster provided researchers with a valuable insight into both bereavement processes and reactions (Lindemann, 1944). There was also evidence to suggest that many survivors suffered from post-traumatic stress, exhibiting symptoms such as flashbacks, panic attacks, extreme tension, breathlessness and an inability to concentrate (Cobb and Lindemann, 1943). Another major disaster of fire, again in the USA, which has been extensively studied for the effects of post-traumatic stress, was the Beverly Hills Supper Club fire of 1977, which resulted in 165 people losing their lives (Green et al, 1983).

There are few studies that have attempted to estimate the extent of PTSD after traumatic incidents in the general population. Those that have, put the rate at between 1 and 3% of the population (Helzer et al, 1987; Davidson et al, 1991). These studies, however, have been conducted in the USA, and, at present, there are no figures for the UK. In disasters, estimates of PTSD tend to be much higher, for example between 22 and 50% (Raphael, 1986; Curran et al, 1990). A recent report from the Home Office Disasters Working Party (Home Office, 1991) estimated that:

> 40%–70% experienced distress in the first month; 24%–40% experienced distress after the first year; 15%–20% experienced chronic levels of anxiety, which remain high for longer than 2 years.

BURN TRAUMA AND PTSD

The literature on burn trauma and PTSD is surprisingly scarce, despite the common occurrence of burn injuries. In the UK, about 900 deaths per year occur as a result of injury by fire, and approximately 15 000 people are admitted to hospital for the same reason (Home Office, 1983). In the USA, it is estimated that approximately 1% annually of the population sustains burns, i.e. approximately 300 000 people, of whom 7000 die (Ochitill, 1984).

It would be hardly surprising if burn injury, which is a painful, frightening and extraordinarily traumatic event, precipitated post-traumatic symptoms in some burns survivors. Andreason and Norris (1972) described transient 'phobic' and 'traumatic' neuroses in many burns survivors in a study that pre-dates DSM–III by at least 8 years. Attempts to predict the development of PTSD in burn trauma have, by and large, been inconclusive. White (1981) found that over one-third of 86 patients admitted for 7 days or more to a Burns Unit, who were followed up 1 year after their accident, had marked psychological sequelae. While this study indicated that pre-morbid vulnerability, i.e. previous history of psychological disorder, could be an important predictor of PTSD, the overwhelming majority of victims who developed post-traumatic stress did not have a past psychiatric history. Other factors found to be important were age, social class and whether patients lived on their own or with large families. There is also no clear relationship between area of injury and the frequency and severity of psychological side-effects. Perry et al (1992) acknowledged limitations in their study of predictors of PTSD after burn injury because of the absence of standardised assessment of psychopathology prior to the trauma. However, despite this shortcoming, high rates of PTSD were found in their sample, even at a 1-year follow-up.

Notable exceptions to the paucity of literature on burn trauma and PTSD are two papers by Courtemanche and Robinow (1989) and Sturgeon et al (1991), which concentrate on specific case examples and treatment strategies used. Sturgeon et al (1991) provide a comprehensive and graphic account of the psychological sequelae and treatment of some of the most severely physically damaged survivors of the King's Cross fire in 1987. Many were troubled by nightmares (invariably involving flames); all described a heightened sense of vigilance in everyday situations, for example crossing the road. They also experienced an intense sense of the frailty of human life and an expectation of further disasters. Many reported flashbacks, disturbed sleep, avoidance of common activities and emotional difficulties on the anniversary of the disaster, all symptoms characteristic of PTSD. The lesson to be learned here is, as Sturgeon et al (1991) conclude, 'that early psychological contact is vital for the emotional and physical well being of the patient in the early stages of recovery'.

The development of PTSD in children post-burn has also been studied, but again the literature is sparse. Stoddard et al (1989) found that when compared with other clinical samples of children, the burn sample had especially high levels of psychiatric disturbance, including PTSD. Some believe that the burn treatment itself becomes a traumatic event, and that, for some children, the longer hospitalisation is extended, with the daily cycle of dressing changes and physiotherapy, the more regressed and withdrawn they become (Sieck, 1990).

While the presence of PTSD does not, in many cases, seem to correlate with the size of the burn, nurses working in this area of critical care should be aware of PTSD as a common and treatable cause of psychological disturbance in the burn patient, especially as the burn injury is often more than an adequate stressor.

ASSESSMENT AND TREATMENT OF PTSD

Assessment of a patient suffering from PTSD can be conducted in a number of ways, but the prime function of the assessment process is to gather enough information to arrive at a decision on what would be the most appropriate form of intervention or treatment. It is quite usual for many people, post-trauma, to experience a number of psychological difficulties, and burn trauma is no exception. It would be erroneous to assume, however, that every burn trauma patient will suffer psychological distress. Therefore, a knowledge and awareness of the symptomatology of PTSD would enable nurses and other professionals to be vigilant for symptoms that persist for at least 1 month post-burn.

Conducting a full assessment may often be beyond the skill and time constraints of many nurses in busy units, but a recognition that there may be problems and a referral for specialist assessment would be an appropriate course of action. The identification of the symptoms indicative of PTSD can, however, be picked up at primary nurse/keyworker level by:

● A knowledge and awareness of the diagnostic criteria for PTSD
● A good relationship and rapport with the patient
● Possession of basic interviewing or counselling skills

Once this has been done, a decision can then be made on whether a referral for specialist assessment and treatment is indicated, or whether the patient would benefit more from some support at ward level. If there is a doubt, a consultation with a psychiatrist, nurse specialist in liaison psychiatry or clinical psychologist would help to clarify the situation and indicate further intervention, if necessary.

Formal assessment can be carried out using structured clinical interviews (SCID) for DSM–IIIR (Spitzer and Williams, 1985) or PSE–10 (Present State Examination, 10th edition), which is in use in the UK (Wing et al, 1990). The aforementioned assessment tools are often more in use for research purposes, and therefore a more likely and equally effective framework of assessment would be a three-systems analysis, which takes the view that anxiety (a significant component of PTSD) is not a unitary concept but is made up of three components:

1. *Autonomic* – the physiological manifestations of anxiety
2. *Behavioural* – the effects of anxiety on the individual's behaviour
3. *Cognitive* – the thoughts an individual experiences when anxious

Each individual will experience different levels of intensity and severity of each of the three systems, and careful assessment can therefore provide valuable information on where to target an intervention as far as PTSD is concerned. Of course, anxiety is not the only presentation; PTSD is often seen in conjunction with other disorders, most commonly depression and substance abuse. Therefore, a wide-ranging assessment focusing down to examine the specific components of PTSD is indicated (for a useful guide see Scott and Stradling, 1992, pp 10–13).

The use of questionnaires or rating scales is a useful adjunct to the assessment process. Those commonly used are the Beck Depression Inventory (BDI) (Beck et al, 1961), the Impact of Events Scale (IES) (Weiss et al, 1984) and the PENN Inventory (Hammarberg, 1992). The latter two rating scales have been specifically devised for sufferers of PTSD. Rating scales are also useful for providing a guide to a patient's progress and highlighting specific areas that may need closer attention.

If a patient is thought to be suffering from PTSD and this is confirmed by formal assessment, the next step is to choose the most appropriate intervention. Almost all treatment for PTSD is psychologically orientated and is aimed at dealing with the range of emotional and behavioural problems outlined earlier. There is evidence that supportive counselling is only of general, rather than specific, use in PTSD sufferers (Duckworth and Charlesworth, 1988), and that the manifestation of PTSD as a specific disorder requires specialised treatment.

Behavioural and cognitive behavioural therapies have, over the past few years, been used successfully in the treatment of PTSD (Frank et al, 1988; Richards and Rose, 1991; Foa et al, 1992). The two most common therapeutic strategies are:

1. Those that help the survivors to 'emotionally process' the memories of the trauma and overcome their avoidances
2. Those that teach survivors additional coping skills and anxiety management techniques

Specific interventions include:

1. *Graded exposure in real life* – This involves the individual confronting previously avoided anxiety-provoking situations, until the anxiety subsides.

2. *Imaginal exposure* – This is a technique that involves direct exposure to memories of the trauma and involves the use of audiotaped material. As with real life exposure, this can also be graded and, with repeated practice, will eventually result in a reduction in anxiety and other related symptoms.

3. *Cognitive therapy* – This often integrates both of the above and is also shown to be effective.

Cognitive therapy is a form of psychotherapy based on a theory of emotional disorders (Beck, 1967). It is a structured form of psychotherapy designed to alleviate symptoms and help patients learn more effective ways of coping with their psychological difficulties. The therapeutic mode of cognitive therapy is problem orientated and semistructured. It is aimed at correcting the combination of psychological and situational problems that may be contributing to the patient's distress. The label 'cognitive therapy' is used because the techniques employed are directed at changing distortions in patients' cognitions. This includes the way in which situations and stressors are appraised, assumptions about themselves, the world and the future, and the beliefs and attitudes that are presumed to increase their vulnerability to emotional problems.

This is a treatment approach based on historical, theoretical and empirical grounds (Blackburn and Davidson, 1990). Many individuals often find that their beliefs and assumptions about themselves, others and their world have been 'shattered' as a result of their experience of trauma (Janoff-Bulman, 1985). The PTSD sufferer's belief in personal invulnerability, their perceptions of the world as meaningful and comprehensible, in their assumptions that other people can be trusted, and in their views of themselves as being a competent and worthwhile person, can be severely challenged. Self-questioning, feelings of insecurity, unworthiness and weakness, and perceptions of threat and danger might be evident. The world might be viewed as threatening, and the likelihood of future recurrence might be seen as high. While this particular feature of PTSD is often experienced by individuals who have been victimised, for example by violent crime, it is also a common feature experienced by anyone who has suffered any form of physical trauma. Therapy aims to address this and helps the sufferer to come to terms with the experience.

All the techniques and strategies described above should always be carried out as individually tailed treatment packages, after thorough assessment and only with the co-operation and collaboration of the patient. The duration of treatment will vary in individual cases; however, average treatment programmes may take place over 12 sessions.

POST-TRAUMATIC STRESS DISORDER – A CASE STUDY

Jane was a 29-year-old mother of two who was referred by the consultant psychiatrist for treatment following a serious accidental explosion at her home 18 months previously. The accident occurred a few days before Christmas. Jane was sitting in her living room by the window wrapping Christmas presents, and her 2-year-old son Robert was playing on the living room carpet. Her husband was momentarily out of the room. Without warning, the back boiler exploded, virtually demolishing the living room and causing severe damage estimated at £12 000.

Robert was seriously injured, suffering a depressed fracture of the frontal lobe of the brain and 12% burns, which required grafting, the areas of most concern being his right forehead (the eyebrow being missing) and the right side of his torso. Jane sustained burns to both legs, mostly superficial, with scattered areas of full thickness. She also received a head injury requiring stitches, sustained when she was hit by flying debris. The accident was serious and dramatic enough to receive headline coverage in the local newspaper, and the senior fire officer attending was quoted as saying, 'If the Lord was on anyone's side, he was on theirs'.

Both mother and son were taken to the local Accident and Emergency Department and then admitted to the sub-regional Burns Unit, where they received treatment. By the time Jane was referred for assessment, she had given birth to a baby girl who was 7 months old, and Robert was making a significant recovery, although he was still being followed up.

Shortly after the explosion, Jane went through a period of clinical depression, which was characterised by appetite and weight loss, diurnal mood variation and bouts of tearfulness. Her irritable bowel syndrome symptoms were exacerbated, and she experienced an increase of migraineous headaches. By the time she was seen by the consultant psychiatrist, she was felt no longer to be suffering from a clinical depression but was nevertheless suffering from marked anxiety reactions, characterised by a variety of symptoms needing specialist psychological intervention.

In the period since the accident, following her initial bout of depression, Jane continued to experience a variety of symptoms, which met the diagnostic criteria for PTSD. She was unable to discuss her son's injuries (which were severe) or her own. She would engage in a variety of avoidance behaviours, characterised by an inability to watch television programmes and read magazines or newspaper articles containing material that served as a reminder of her own experiences. If confronted with any of the above situations, she would experience marked symptoms of panic, for example palpitations, tremors, headaches and sweating. This would then have a significant effect on her mood, leading to irritability and tearfulness. Jane also exhibited a significant degree of obsessional behaviour, which resulted in a preoccupation with and frequent checking of electrical appliances, such as the gas fire and the cooker. This would often cause her enough anxiety to lead her back to the house more than once after she had left, to make numerous physical checks.

Her relationship with her husband was also put under considerable strain, and she found that she was becoming overprotective and overconcerned with her son's welfare, the latter inevitably having implications for his future psychological development and well-being. Jane also found that she was unable to discuss the accident with anybody she might meet on a casual or social basis, the reason being that, as she had never adequately 'emotionally processed' her experience, she would inevitably become extremely distressed and consequently withdraw from the situation.

Jane was also experiencing bouts of anxiety and depression, which were triggered by the continuing treatment Robert required because of his injuries. Both she and her husband (not unnaturally) found his continuing care a constant source of worry and a strain. Jane also had marked concern about Robert's ability to integrate with other children, owing to the cosmetic nature of his injuries, and she worried that this might cause some problems at school and then in later life; to some extent, these concerns were not without substance. Jane also experienced feelings of guilt and anger about the incident and her part in Robert's aftercare. She felt that she could have done more at the time of the accident to help to remove him from the scene of the explosion. She recalled that at the time of the accident, she made every attempt to try to reach her son, but was so bewildered, shocked and frightened that she could not locate him in the room, being in darkness and also handicapped by her own injuries. Consequently, she made for the nearest chink of light and stumbled free to get help. She began to see this as an act of selfishness rather than the only course of action open to her at the time.

At the assessment, she was given a rationale for treatment and a fairly detailed explanation of what a cognitive behavioural approach to her difficulties would entail. While she was not unnaturally apprehensive, she was nevertheless extremely motivated to engage in treatment, as she felt she was considerably debilitated by her symptoms. She was also extremely concerned that her behaviour would begin to affect Robert adversely. Before treatment commenced, her husband was seen and his aid enlisted as co-therapist. Her health visitor was also contacted and informed of the treatment planned.

Jane's treatment consisted of the following components:

1. *Cognitive anxiety management training* – This consisted of a variety of strategies that were aimed at enhancing her coping skills, including the use of relaxation therapy, teaching Jane diaphragmatic breathing exercises and educating her about PTSD and all the contributing factors that led to the development and maintenance of her emotional and behavioural problems. She was also taught the principles of exposure therapy and how to measure her anxiety.

2. *Exposure in vivo (real life)* – This involved Jane facing up to a number of situations that she had previously avoided. As there were a variety of situations, the programme was graded, and Jane devised her own hierarchy of feared situations. As mentioned earlier, exposure is a technique whereby individuals have to confront feared situations until their anxiety reduces to a manageable level. This process is known as habituation and is used commonly with many phobic problems. Jane inevitably found this technique quite difficult; sessions would sometimes last up to 4 hours and involve a significant degree of discomfort and hard work on her part.

3. *Exposure in imagination* – This component was very similar to that outlined above, but concerned exposing Jane to a variety of distressing thoughts and traumatic imagery concerning the accident. She was asked to describe it in the first person, and present tense, as though it were actually occurring. This was then audiotaped, and she would then listen to this for as much as five or six times a week, replaying the tape on each occasion until she noticed a reduction in her anxiety. By the seventh session, habituation had taken place and she found that she was getting 'bored' and that her mind was 'wandering', evidence, therefore, that the traumatic imagery and memories were no longer as potent.

4. *Cognitive restructuring* – This involved Jane keeping a detailed diary of her thoughts and emotions throughout therapy, and was specifically aimed at getting her to emotionally 'reprocess' her traumatic experience. She was eventually able to challenge and modify her beliefs about not having acted more appropriately at the time of the incident, and was able to accept that she did everything humanly possible at the time and in the circumstances.

Jane had received 14 sessions, totalling approximately 24 hours of therapy time when she was discharged. At discharge, Jane had improved by approximately 80% in all areas, as indicated by all rating scales and measures used. She was able to discuss the accident without undue anxiety and also discuss the injuries that Robert had received. She was also able to read newspaper reports about her accident and watch television documentaries or read previously disturbing newspaper and magazine articles. Jane also reported that she was far less irritable at home, experienced fewer significant fluctuations in mood and felt that she had, by and large, come to terms with her experience. She worked extremely hard in treatment and was highly motivated throughout, which was an undoubted contributing factor to the significant progress she had made. Jane was seen up to the year after the end of treatment for follow-up, and she had continued to maintain her progress. Robert had continued to improve, and while it was felt that he might have some difficulties with language and concentration after the accident, he was making excellent progress at school, was socialising well and had many friends. It was clear that despite his injuries, which were far more serious, he was psychologically unaffected by the accident.

SUMMARY

As highlighted earlier, many, but not all, burn victims develop PTSD. Good physical and psychological nursing, remedial and medical care will often be enough to allow the majority of individuals to come to terms with their trauma and deal with it appropriately. In the light of the evidence, however, PTSD may manifest itself in many individuals who suffer a burn injury. Other factors, for example the part that significant others may have played in the trauma and the impact this will have had on all concerned, also need to be taken into account.

Assessment, perhaps at an informal level at first, followed by a more thorough formal assessment process, is essential. Sensitivity on the part of nursing, remedial and medical staff is of paramount importance in terms of gaining the patient's confidence and trust, thus allowing him to disclose traumatic and painful memories. Many individuals suffering from PTSD can feel set apart from others because of their symptoms and their experience. They may be hesitant to discuss events surrounding their trauma, and may even report fears that they may be going 'mad'. Therefore, a sound knowledge base is extremely important in order that their thoughts, feelings and behaviours can be acknowledged and 'normalised' in the context of their experience.

A number of effective treatment strategies have been developed for individuals suffering PTSD, and access to treatment should be sought and made available at an early stage of the disorder. Treatment will not only diminish the effects of this particularly disabling disorder, but also encourage and allow for the most complete rehabilitation possible. Nurses and remedial staff are often best placed to identify the disorder in its infancy and seek consultation and supervision as to further intervention strategies.

Artz (1979) once suggested that 'The need for psychiatric assistance [in the care of burn patients] should be rare'. There is now a wealth of literature to confirm psychological disturbance following burn injury (Wallace and Lees, 1988; Watkins et al, 1988). Knowledge of PTSD as a specific psychological sequela of burn trauma is becoming increasingly common, mainly through greater awareness and reporting of the disorder in the psychological and psychiatric literature. It is also clear that, in the arena of psychological care, it is an area that warrants continued empirical scrutiny, especially as psychological assessment, treatment and evaluation are an essential component of the overall care and rehabilitation of the burn victim.

References

American Psychiatric Association (1980) *Diagnostic and Statistical Manual of Mental Disorders*. Washington: American Psychiatric Association.

American Psychiatric Association (1987) *Diagnostic and Statistical Manual of Mental Disorders*, 3rd edn (revised). Washington: American Psychiatric Association.

American Psychiatric Association (1994) *Diagnostic and Statistical Manual of Mental Disorders*, 4th edn Washington: American Psychiatric Association.

Andreason NJC and Norris AS (1972) Long term adjustment and adaptation mechanisms in severely burned adults. *Journal of Nervous and Mental Disease* **154:** 352–362.

Artz CP (1979) Psychological considerations. In: Artz CP, Moncrief JA and Pruitt BA (eds) *Burns: A Team Approach*, pp 35–37. Philadelphia: WB Saunders.

Beck AT (1967) *Depression: Clinical, Experimental and Theoretical Aspects*. New York: Hoeber.

Beck AT, Ward DH, Mendelson M et al (1961) An inventory for measuring depression. *Archives of General Psychiatry* **4:** 561–571.

Blackburn I and Davidson K (1990) *Cognitive Therapy for Depression and Anxiety*. Oxford: Blackwell.

Blanchard EB, Kolb LC, Pallmeyer TP and Gerardi RJ (1982) A psychological study of Post Traumatic Stress Disorder in Vietnam veterans. *Psychiatric Quarterly* **54:** 220–229.

Burgess WW and Holmstrom LL (1974) Rape trauma syndrome. *American Journal of Psychiatry* **131**(9): 981–986.

Cobb S and Lindermann E (1943) Neuropsychiatric observations on the Cocoanut Grove fire. *Annals of Surgery* **117:** 814–824.

Curran PS, Bell P, Murray G et al (1990) Psychological consequences of the Enniskillen bombing. *British Journal of Psychiatry* **156:** 479–482.

Courtemanche DJ and Robinow O (1989) The recognition and treatment of the Post Traumatic Stress Disorder in the burn victim. *Journal of Burn Care and Rehabilitation* **10**(3): 247–250.

Daly RJ (1983). Samuel Pepys and Post Traumatic Stress Disorder. *British Journal of Psychiatry* **143:** 64–68.

Davidson JRT, Hughes D, Blazer DG and George LK (1991) Post Traumatic Stress Disorder in the community: an epidemiological study. *Psychological Medicine* **21:** 713–721.

Duckworth DH and Charlesworth A (1988) The human side of disaster. *Policing* **4:** 194–210.

Foa EB, Rothbaum BO, Riggs DS and Murdoch TB (1992) Treatment of Post Traumatic Stress Disorder in rape victims: a comparison between cognitive behavioural procedures and counselling. *Journal of Counselling and Clinical Psychology* **59:** 715–723.

Frank E, Anderson B, Stewart BD et al (1988) Efficacy of cognitive behaviour therapy and systematic de-sensitisation in the treatment of rape trauma. *Behaviour Therapy* **19:** 403–420.

Green BL, Grace MC, Lindy JD et al (1983) Levels of functional impairment following a civilian disaster: the Beverly Hills Supper Club fire. *Journal of Counsulting and Clinical Psychology* **51:** 573–580.

Hammarberg M (1992) PENN Inventory for Post Traumatic Stress Disorder: psychometric properties. *Psychological Assessment: A Journal of Consulting and Clinical Psychology* **4:** 67–76.

Helzer JE, Robbins LN and McEvoy L (1987) Post Traumatic Stress Disorder in the general population: findings from the epidemiological catchment area survey. *New England Journal of Medicine* **317:** 1630–1634.

Hodgkinson PE (1990) The Zeebrugge disaster. III. Psychological care in the UK. *Disaster Management* **2:** 131–134.

Home Office (1983) *Fire Statistics*. London: HMSO.

Home Office (1991) *Disasters, Planning for a Caring Response*. London: HMSO.

Janoff-Bulman R (1985) The aftermath of victimization: rebuilding shattered assumptions. In: Figley CR (ed.) *Trauma and its Wake: The Study and Treatment of Post Traumatic Stress Disorder*, pp 15–35. New York: Bruner Mazel.

Latham R and Matthews W (1970–83) *The Diary of Samuel Pepys*, 11 vols. London: Bell & Hyman.

Lindemann E (1944) Symptomatology and management of acute grief. *American Journal of Psychiatry* **101:** 141–148.

Ochitill H (1984) Psychiatric consultation to the Burns Unit: the psychiatrist's perspective. *American Journal of Psychosomatic Medicine* **25:** 697–702.

Perry S, Difede J, Musngi G et al (1992) Predictors of Post Traumatic Stress Disorder after burn injury. *American Journal of Psychiatry* **149**(7): 931–935.

Raphael B (1986) *When Disaster Strikes: A Handbook for the Caring Professions*. London: Hutchinson.

Richards DA and Rose JS (1991) Exposure therapy for Post Traumatic Stress Disorder: four case studies. *British Journal of Psychiatry* **158**: 836–840.

Rothbaum BO, Foa EB, Riggs, DS et al (1992) A prospective examination of Post Traumatic Stress Disorder in rape victims. *Journal of Traumatic Stress* **5**: 455–475.

Scott MJ and Stradling, SG (1992) *Counselling for Post Traumatic Stress Disorder*. London: Sage.

Sieck HS (1990) Post Traumatic Stress Disorder. *Journal of Burn and Rehabilitation* **11**(1): 96 (letter; comment).

Spitzer RL and Williams JBW (1985). *Structured Clinical Interview for DSM–II–R: Patient Version*. New York: Biometrics Research Department, New York State Psychiatric Institute.

Stoddard TJ, Norman DK and Murphy JM (1989) A diagnostic outcome study of children and adolescents with severe burns. *Journal of Trauma* **29**(4): 471–477.

Sturgeon D, Rosser R and Shoenberg P (1991) The Kings Cross fire. Part 2. The psychological injuries. *Burns* **17**(1): 10–13.

Trimble MR (1985) Post Traumatic Stress Disorder; history of a concept. In: Figley CR (ed.) *Trauma and its Wake: The Study and Treatment of Post Traumatic Stress Disorder*, p 5214. New York: Brunner Mazel.

Wallace LM and Lees J (1988) A psychological follow-up study of adult patients discharged from a Burns Unit. *Burns Journal* **14**: 39–45.

Watkins PN, Cook EL, May SR and Ehleben CM (1988) Psychological stages in adaptation following burn injury. A method for facilitation of psychological recovery of burn victims. *Journal of Burn Care and Rehabilitation* **9**: 376–384.

Weiss D, Horowitz MJ and Wilner N (1984) The stress response rating scale: a clinician's measure for rating the response to various life events. *British Journal of Clinical Psychology* **23**: 205–215.

White AC (1981) *Psychiatric study of severely injured burn victims*. MD thesis, University of Birmingham.

Wing JK, Babor T, Brugha et al (1990) SCAN: Schedules for Clinical Assessment in Neuro Psychiatry. *Archives of General Psychiatry* **47**: 589–593.

15

Staff Support
on the Burns Unit

At present, there are constant and often significant changes in the modern NHS, and the notions of stress and crisis will be familiar, if uncomfortable, themes for many nurses and allied professions. Thus, many nurses have not only to live with the uncertainty of change on an organisational basis, but also to cope with demanding environmental and professional situations. While no health-care professional is immune to these pressures, there is evidence that suggests that many areas of nursing, particularly those areas we think of as critical care environments, for example Accident and Emergency, Intensive Care and Burns Units, are often the most vulnerable to stress, and in need of much support (Huckaby and Jagla, 1979; Bishop, 1983; Jacobson, 1983; von Baeyer and Krause, 1983).

The questions that invariably spring to mind are: are staff in these areas supported, and, if so, what is the nature of that support and who provides it? This chapter is primarily concerned with the development and maintenance of staff support on a subregional Burns Unit. There are, however, a number of other issues that are of relevance when discussing the nature and provision of staff support in this and other areas of critical care nursing. Therefore, the main issues under discussion will be:

- The nature of stress, the importance of the role of cognitions (thoughts) and their influence on emotions and behaviour
- The case for staff support
- A comprehensive and flexible model for staff support on a Burns Unit

THE NATURE OF STRESS

Many explanations of stress tend to be somewhat simplistic, in that they do not allow for variations in individual circumstances or events. Since the early 1980s, much more sophisticated models of stress have evolved, thus giving us a greater understanding not only of the nature of stress, but also of how to deal with it more effectively. Lazarus (1981) noted that individuals are not mere victims of stress, but that two factors in particular determine the nature of stress. These are:

1. How they appraise stressful events (primary appraisal)

2. How they appraise their coping resources and options (secondary appraisal)

The individual's appraisal processes influence the relationship or transaction between the individual and the social environment, which is constantly changing. Meichenbaum (1985) also proposes the notion that stress and coping are transactional in nature. The concept of stress has been defined in a variety of ways. Some researchers have defined stress as a condition of the environment, for example work stressors, raising children or the stress of competition. According to this view, stress represents a set of external forces impinging upon the individual or the group. Another common view of stress relates to the individual's response when placed in a challenging or threatening environment.

At this point, it would be appropriate to examine the influential role played by an individual's cognitions (thoughts and images) and feelings, experienced before, during and after an event. Given that cognitions influence stress, it is worth considering this concept in more detail. The concept of cognitions can be divided into three different areas, namely:

- Cognitive events
- Cognitive processes
- Cognitive structures

Cognitive Events

Cognitive events are conscious, identifiable thoughts and images. Beck (1976) describes these as automatic thoughts; they invariably appear in shorthand form, are almost always unquestioned and believed, are often expressed as *'shoulds'*, *'oughts' or 'musts'*, are relatively idiosyncratic, and are difficult to turn off. They also appear plausible and valid. Meichenbaum (1977) has described such cognitive events as a form of internal dialogue, the sort of 'little conversations' one has with oneself, either prior to, during or after an event. This dialogue incorporates, among other things, attributions, expectations, self-evaluation and related or irrelevant thoughts and images.

The nature and content of such cognitive events can significantly influence how one feels and behaves. Therefore, individuals under stress tend to become self-focused and often display a variety of self-defeating thoughts and feelings, which will further increase emotional disturbances. Thus, individuals prone to stress are loaded to make one-sided, extreme, absolute and global judgments, often tending to personalise events and engage in cognitive distortions, such as polarisation (black and white dichotomous reasoning), magnification and exaggeration (overemphasis on the most negative possibilities in a given situation), and overgeneralisation. These distortions often occur in an automatic, unconscious fashion (Beck, 1984).

Cognitive Processes

The term 'cognitive processes' refers to the ways in which we automatically or unconsciously process information, including how we store, retrieve and search for information. These processes shape our schemata, i.e. our beliefs and assumptions about ourselves, others and our world. Most of the time, we do not think about the way we think or how we appraise situations, how we selectively attend and recall events or how we selectively seek information consistent with our beliefs. For example, individuals who feel strongly that the world *should* be fair are likely to be hypervigilant for signs of potential injustice and misread events as personal slights. This would, in turn, affect their mood and behaviour.

Cognitive Structures

'Cognitive structures' encompasses the tacit assumptions, beliefs and meanings that influence habitual ways of construing oneself and the world. Cognitive structures can be thought of as schemata, which are mental organisations of experience. These are the way in which an individual interprets his world and makes sense of experiences. Therefore, the way in which we interpret, perceive, appraise and evaluate events significantly influences our emotions and behaviour. The work of Beck (1984) indicates that stressful life events can trigger such schemata, and views such schemata as specific sensitive areas or specific emotional vulnerabilties that result in individuals' predilections to overreact. Such hypersensitivities or cognitive structures act as templates that influence the way in which situations are appraised and that guide cognitive processes, emotions and behaviours.

The work of Lazarus, Beck, Meichenbaum and others has made a significant contribution to our understanding of anxiety and the nature of stress. Most importantly, their work has given substance to the notion that high levels of stress are largely brought about by an individual's interpretation of an event, rather than the event per se.

Another important factor in our understanding of the nature of stress is the role played by life events. A considerable amount of evidence, stemming from the work of Holmes and Rahe (1967), indicates that certain life events that cause change increase an individual's vulnerability to stress-related illness. These life events involve change of some kind, for example in health, family relationships, economic and living conditions, education, religion and social affairs. They range in seriousness from major life crises, such as the death of a partner, to relatively minor events, such as going on holiday or receiving a parking ticket.

The only difficulty with this early attempt to classify and describe life events (even though it holds much relevance today) is that it is unidimensional and deals only with stress. As mentioned previously, cognitive appraisal is important, as perceptions of a stressful event may vary from one individual to another. An important point that needs to be made here is that one individual's life event becomes another's. This is especially relevant in areas of critical care nursing, for example the Burns Unit, where nurses have to contend not only with high levels of stress caused by distressing procedures, but also with a variety of psychosocial factors. A significant proportion of burn injuries occurs in the context of stressful life events. Adults with a burn injury often have psychiatric conditions that increase their susceptibility to injury. Many victims are also single, unemployed and from disadvantaged backgrounds, which increases their vulnerability (Noyes et al, 1979). A number come from disturbed family backgrounds, in which unemployment, poor housing and relationship problems may complicate the situation (Kolman, 1983).

In view of the above, many nurses can be and very often are, touched by the lives of the individuals they nurse. A high level of emotional and personal involvement, rather than being viewed in negative terms, should be supported, and a framework provided whereby that support can be accessed on a personal and professional level. The nature of support needs to be tangible and flexible in order to respond to the demands that staff face in such a challenging environment.

THE CASE FOR STAFF SUPPORT

Many studies have provided evidence that nurses in specialised areas are vulnerable to stress (Shubin, 1978; Maslach, 1981; Jacobsen, 1983; Beaver et al, 1986). Bailey (1985) suggests that nurses and medical staff are often more at risk than are those they care for. Melia (1987) notes the main concern for many nurses as being issues of control or power regarding decisions pertinent to care. Individuals who feel they have no control over what is happening to them or what they do have been found to experience high levels of stress (Weiss, 1972; Cohen, 1980). There is further evidence that individuals who think they have no control over events can learn to become helpless. This 'learned helplessness' in turn leads to stress (Seligman, 1975).

Nurses are often faced with making decisions of enormous responsibility without the immediate support of a team and without adequate supervision. Another area of stress in nursing is in the professional arena, in which nurses may feel undervalued or taken for granted. In the present climate, competition for employment is intense, which is inevitably a source of tension and dissatisfaction. Inadequate and poor communication can lead to misunderstandings and misinterpretation of intentions and behaviour, thus creating an environment in which the stress is constantly perpetuated because opportunities are never taken to resolve outstanding, organisational and interpersonal issues (Cassee, 1975). Stress in the area of critical care nursing is an acknowledged concern, and there is recent evidence in the literature to highlight this (Llewelyn, 1989; Wright, 1991). It would be pertinent at this point to move on to examine a specific example of staff support and discuss a number of issues of relevance, in an attempt to answer the questions posed in the introduction to this chapter.

STAFF SUPPORT ON THE BURNS UNIT –
A WORKING MODEL

It is not the intention here to discuss at any length the mechanics of setting up a support group. That is comprehensively covered by a number of authors (Burnard,

1991; Nichols and Jenkinson, 1991; Wright, 1991) and worthy of scrutiny for those readers considering either setting up or leading a support group. Llewelyn (1989) makes a good point in advising caution in applying some of the techniques advocated, as they can be beneficial if chosen as individual coping strategies, but can be counterproductive if imposed on people without consideration or regard for individual circumstances.

Antebi (1993) has described the work of the psychiatrist on the Burns Unit and the setting up of a consultation–liaison service. The model for staff meetings and support was multidisciplinary (excluding medical staff – no reasons are given other than to say that they approached the psychiatrist separately for discussions). The meetings were held weekly; the content was decided by staff and was usually based around teaching on a specific psychological or psychiatric problem, followed by discussion of 'problem' patients. No pressure was exerted for staff to attend, although there appeared to be a core group of regular attenders.

Psychiatrists at registrar and senior registrar levels rotate, so consistency and continuity may be a problem, as may their availability in any given circumstances. The unit described in Antebi's (1993) paper still has support in the form of a senior registrar, but regular input is provided on a weekly basis by the author (a senior clinical nurse specialist in cognitive behavioural psychotherapy), and the model is flexible by intent, providing a forum for individual supervision, consultation or support (group). Staff on the unit (at the time of writing), work 'long' days, for example 12-hour shifts, as a result of a consensus decision, and therefore attendance at a group is variable; however, it averages five staff plus students.

This input, which by its nature is a consultation–liaison psychiatry service, has five main features:

1. *Consultation* – which could encompass a wide range of activities, for example training or advice and guidance on specific or general issues.

2. *Supervision* – for assessment or intervention.

3. *Staff support* – either individual or group. This could include case discussion and emerging themes.

4. *Teaching* – on specific psychological problems and their management.

5. *Clinical input* – as and where appropriate, to patients who require therapy or counselling. This could also be purely for assessment, to establish or clarify a psychological care plan.

Certain practical problems have to be acknowledged and worked around, given the intrinsic nature of the environment. Therefore the basic format or ground rules of the group setting are as follows:

1. Confidentiality is paramount, especially if the group at any point deals with the personal issues of those present at the time.

2. Interruptions are, within reason, acceptable (given the demands of the unit).

Case
Death of a child from 85% BSA burns

Theme 1
Junior staff members' first experience of a severe injury –
What ways are there of dealing with this?

Theme 2
Ethical dilemma/issues discussed,
e.g. Is getting involved purely spectatoring or
a valuable learning experience?

Theme 3
The role of students in a case like this –
What are the issues regarding their support and preparation?

Theme 4
Discussion of organisational stressors and areas of conflict/responsibility

General discussion/feedback of the emergent themes and
also thoughts, feelings, reactions
and lessons learnt

Fig 15.1   Support group – example of case discussion and emergent themes

3.   Staff members will not be discussed in their absence.

4.   Managerial and organisational aspects will be discussed only if all those concerned are present.

5.   The format of the group is flexible, but the main focus is the presentation of a case history and the discussion of any emergent themes (Figure 15.1)

6.   Specific teaching requests can be made and planned in advance

In addition to the above, other features, for example problem-solving (Sobel and Worden, 1981) and psychological debriefing (Dyregrov, 1989), can be built into or form an essential part of staff support.

Common to many problem-solving programmes is a formula that involves the following steps and is useful for case management:

- Define the stress or stress reaction to be problem-solved
- Establish realistic goals
- Generate a wide range of alternative solutions
- Imagine or consider others' reactions to similar stressors

- Evaluate the pros and cons of each proposed solution, and rank solutions in order, from the least to the most practical and desirable
- Possibly rehearse chosen strategies
- Try out the most acceptable and feasible solution
- Reconsider the original problem in the light of the attempt at problem-solving
- Expect some failures, but reward oneselves for effort

Another important aspect of staff support is 'Critical Incident Stress Debriefing' (CISD) (Mitchell, 1983) or 'Psychological Debriefing' (Dyregrov, 1989). These two terms are often used to describe the same process, but the former is in more common usage. CISD is now widely used with emergency service personnel, the armed forces and in a variety of situations where individuals or groups have been exposed to a traumatic event. This is a process that enables either individuals or a group to deal with the aftermath of traumatic events. Given the nature of the work of a Burns Unit and of the circumstances of many of the injuries seen, debriefing, when used appropriately, could be an invaluable tool in the repertoire of a support group facilitator. The aim of a debriefing is to minimise the occurrence of unnecessary psychological suffering after a traumatic incident, by allowing the ventilation of emotions, reactions and experiences. Although invariably made available for groups, it can also be extremely helpful for individuals who have been involved in any way in a serious trauma, for example staff involved in a major incident or dealing with seriously injured adults and children. For a useful review of prevention and intervention in critical incident stress, see Mitchell and Dyregrov (1993).

However, given that CISD/psychological debriefing is in wide use at present the ongoing debate concerning its effectiveness is worthy of mention in this context, especially if some readers may have had experience of the process. Recently there have been calls for more research into its application, using randomised controlled trials (Raphael et al, 1985; Bisson and Deahl, 1994). There appear to be two camps, those who believe that CISD is effective in preventing post traumatic reactions and post traumatic stress disorder (PTSD) and those that cast doubt on its efficacy until further evaluative studies are done. Of a review of 36 papers on CISD/psychological debriefing published between 1993 and 1996, 31 were purely descriptive. The others reported outcome data, but there were considerable inconsistencies and difficulties with the methodology. The very nature of CISD, and its application after a traumatic experience, raises ethical implications with relation to research into its effectiveness. The most obvious example of a common methodological shortcoming is the absence of a control group as highlighted by a recent review of CISD research (Bisson and Deahl, 1994), though this in itself raises ethical and legal issues given the now relatively widespread use of the technique with groups such as emergency services personnel. There are a number of other methodological issues that are worthy of consideration, but in the main, the lack of standardisation in the debriefing process itself is something that needs to be addressed in any future research. Mitchell's (1983) original 7 stage CISD model has (not surprisingly) been adapted to take account of the specific needs of a group undergoing the debriefing (Armstrong et al, 1991). Inevitably, these subtle differences in method and process introduces a variety of confounding variables, which has significant implications for the methodology of any outcome studies or evaluative research into CISD.

At the time of writing a few studies are under way with the aim of evaluating the effects and impact of CISD on the development of psychological sequelae following exposure to traumatic events. Therefore the jury is still out. This author however, is prepared to admit to subscribing to the principles and practice of CISD and whilst acknowledging some doubts as to whether as an intervention it prevents the development of PTSD, is more inclined to the belief that it leads primarily to *earlier help seeking*. If this indeed is found to be true, then the psycho-educational benefits alone of the CISD process should be actively utilised, within a supportive framework.

Finally, it would be wholly fitting to conclude this chapter on staff support by discussing the extremely important role of the facilitator. It is the author's view that facilitators should be trained and experienced in psychological models of care and involved in clinical practice. They should possess counselling or psycho-therapy skills in both group and individual settings. They should also have a knowledge, in general terms, of the clinical environment in which support is to be provided, for example the client group, the types of psychosocial and psychological problems experienced, and an awareness of relevant literature and research. A technical knowledge is not always essential, especially if the facilitator is only providing staff support; however, if he is to fulfil a number of other functions, as mentioned earlier, some knowledge is desirable. This can be gained by attendance at ward reviews and spending time with staff in clinical situations.

The choice of facilitator for a support group can be difficult. Given the variety of counselling and psychotherapeutic models available, one way to arrive at the decision would be to arrange meetings with possible facilitators and members of the ward or unit. Staff could then have the opportunity to discuss their needs and learn about the counselling and psychotherapeutic orientation of the prospective facilitator. The choice will inevitably be determined by the style, orientation and personality of the individual and whether the staff feel he would meet their needs. Some models of staff support and methods such as those suggested by Burnard (1991) may be acceptable to some but not others. A framework of support and supervision is also essential (albeit even at peer level) for anyone engaged in consultation–liaison work, especially as this is a growing area of need and is still in a relatively embryonic stage of development in nursing (Tunmore, 1994; Regel and Davies, 1995; Regel, 1995).

The notion of staff support is therefore starting to be recognised as an impor-tant area of need in many challenging critical care environments. A further acknowledgement is that the demands of today's rapidly changing NHS and the pressures created by those changes gives the case for providing a framework for staff support even greater urgency. In the caring professions, we are often notori-ous for not looking after those who provide the care. In a recent report published by the Health and Safety Executive, Cox (1993) argues that at least part of the effects of any stress management programme (whatever it's nature) is due to the way they alter workers' perceptions of and attitudes to their organisations and hence organisational culture. He also argues that poor organisational culture might be associated with an experience of stress, while a good organisational culture might weaken the effects of stress on health. Therefore senior managers and clinicians should take a leaf out of the book of successful corporate organisations (especially in the new 'corporate culture' of the NHS) and adopt a relatively simple rule: Look after your staff and they become more productive and cost effective, not to mention a more contented workforce.

References

Antebi D (1993) The psychiatrist on the burns unit. *Burns*, **19**(1): 43–46.

Armstrong K, O'Callaghan W and Marmer CR (1991) Debriefing Red Cross disaster personnel: the multiple stressor debriefing model. *Journal of Traumatic Stress* **4**: 581–593.

Bailey RD (1985) *Coping with Stress in Caring.* Oxford: Blackwell Scientific.

Beaver RC, Sharp ES and Cotonis GA (1986) Burnout experienced by nurse-midwives. *Journal of Nurse Midwifery* **31**: 3–15.

Beck A (1976) *Cognitive Therapy and the Emotional Disorders.* New York: International Universities Press.

Beck A (1984) Cognitive approaches to stress. In: Woolfolk R and Lehrer P (eds) *Principles and Practice of Stress Management*, New York: Guilford Press.

Bishop V (1983) Stress in the intensive care unit. *Occupational Health* **35**(12): 537–543.

Bisson JI and Deahl MP (1994) Psychological debriefing and prevention of post traumatic stress – more research is needed. *British Journal of Psychiatry.* **165**: 717–720.

Burnard P (1991) *Coping with Stress in the Health Professions – A Practical Guide.* London: Chapman & Hall.

Cassee E (1975) Therapeutic behaviour, hospital culture and communication. In: Cox C and Mead A (eds) *A Sociology of Medical Practice*, London: Collier Macmillan.

Cohen S (1980) After effects of stress on human performance and social behaviour: a review of research and theory. *Psychological Bulletin* **87**: 578–604.

Cox T (1993) *Stress research and sress management: putting theory to work.* Health and Safety Executive Contract Research Report No. 61/1993. HMSO: London.

Dyregrov A (1989) Caring for workers in disaster situations: psychological debriefing. *Disaster Management* **2**: 25–30.

Holmes TH and Rahe RH (1967) The Social Readjustment Rating Scale. *Journal of Psychosomatic Research* **11**: 213–218.

Huckaby LMD and Jagla B (1979) Nurses' stress factors in the intensive care unit. *Journal of Nursing Administration* **9**(2): 21.

Jacobsen SF (1983) Nurses' stress in intensive and nonintensive care units. In: Jacobsen SF and McGrath HM (eds) *Nurses under Stress*, John Chichester: Wiley & Sons.

Kolman P (1983) The incidence of psychopathology in burned adult patients – a critical review. *Journal of Burn Care and Rehabilitation* **416**: 430–436.

Lazarus R (1981) The stress and coping paradigm. In: Eisdorfer C (ed.) *Models for Clinical Psychopathology*, Englewood Cliffs, NJ: Prentice Hall.

Llewelyn S (1989) Caring: the cost to nurses and relatives. In: Broome A (ed.) *Health Psychology – Processes and Applications*, London: Chapman & Hall.

Maslach C (1981) *Burnout: The Cost of Caring.* New York: Prentice Hall.

Meichenbaum D (1977) *Cognitive Behaviour Modification: An Integrative Approach.* New York: Plenum/Press.

Meichenbaum D (1985) *Stress Inoculation Training.* New York: Pergamon Press.

Melia K (1987) Everyday ethics for nurses. *Nursing Times* **83**(3): 28–32.

Mitchell JT (1983) When disaster strikes . . . the critical incident debriefing. *Journal of the Emergency Services.* **8**: 36–39.

Mitchell JT and Dyregrov A (1993) Traumatic stress in disaster workers and emergency personnel. In JP Wilson and B. Raphael (Eds), *International handbook of traumatic stress syndromes*, pp 905–914. New York: Plenum Press.

Nichols K and Jenkinson J (1991) *Leading a Support Group*. London: Chapman & Hall.

Noyes R Frye SJ, Slymen DJ and Canter A (1979) Stressful life events and burn injuries. *The Journal of Trauma* **19(3):** 141–144.

Parkinson F (1993) *Post Trauma Stress*. London: Insight Press.

Raphael B, Meldrum L and McFarlane AC (1995) Does debriefing after psychological trauma work? *British Medical Journal*, **310**: 1479–1480.

Regel S and Davies J (1995) The future of mental health nurses in Liaison Psychiatry. *British Journal of Nursing* **4**: 1052–1056.

Regel S (1995) The role and contribution of mental health nurses in Liaison Psychiatry. *Proceedings of 21st International Conference on Mental Health Nursing, 'Celebrating a New Era'*. Canberra, Australia.

Seligman MEP (1975) *Helplessness*. San Francisco: Freeman.

Shubin S (1978) Burnout: the professional hazard you face in nursing. *Nursing* **8**: 22–27.

Sobel H and Worden J (1981) *Helping Cancer Patients Cope: A Problem Solving Intervention for Health Care Professionals*. New York: BMA/Guilford Press.

Tunmore R (1994) Encouraging collaboration. *Nursing Times* **20**: 66–67.

von Baeyer C and Krause L (1983) Effectiveness of stress management training for nurses working in a burn treatment unit. *International Journal of Psychiatry in Medicine*, **13:** 13–125.

Weiss JM (1972) Influence of psychological variables on stress induced pathology. In: Porter R and Knight (eds) *Physiology, Emotion and Psychosomatic Illness*, New York: American Elsevier.

Wright B (1991) *Sudden Death – Intervention Skills for the Caring Professions*. Edinburgh: Churchill Livingstone.

Index

Page numbers in **bold** type refer to main discussions; those in *italics* refer to figures and tables.